Health Care
Consumers
in the
1990s

Other Books by Richard Thomas

The Demography of Health and Health Care
(with Louis G. Pol; Plenum)

Desktop Marketing: Lessons from America's Best
(with Russell J. Kirchner; American Demographics Books)

The Sociology of Mental Illness: An Annotated Bibliography
(Garland)

HEALTH CARE CONSUMERS IN THE 1990S

Richard K. Thomas

AMERICAN DEMOGRAPHICS BOOKS
ITHACA, NEW YORK

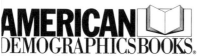

A Division of American Demographics, Inc.
127 West State Street, Ithaca, NY 14850
Telephone: 607-273-6343

Executive Editor: Diane Crispell
Associate Publisher: James Madden
Assistant Editors: Kathleen Brandenburg, Mary Colella
Book Design and Composition: Anne Kilgore
Dust Jacket Production: Rebecca Wilson

This publication is designed to provide accurate and authoritative information in regard to the subject matter covered. It is sold with the understanding that the publisher is not engaged in rendering legal, accounting, or other professional services. If legal advice or other expert assistance is required, the services of a competent professional should be sought.

ISBN 0-936889-19-5
Library of Congress Catalog Number 92-55060

Cataloging In Publication Data
Thomas Richard K. 1944-

Contents

. . . .

FOREWORD

. . . .

THE PAST five years have seen major changes in the U.S. health care system. Competition for patients has intensified in all sectors of the industry, including medical groups, hospitals, and alternative health care organizations. In the face of this increasing competition, many health care providers have adopted the principles of total quality management (TQM) to provide attractive services to consumers.

A key element to succeeding in today's complex health care environment lies in understanding those all-important consumers—who they are, what they want, and how they buy. This new book by Richard Thomas offers important insights into these questions, and is an invaluable resource to anyone involved in the health care industry who wants to better understand the marketplace. It focuses on the health care customer and consumption of health care more clearly and in a more current fashion than any other book available today.

Health Care Consumers in the 1990s should be required reading for anyone trying to integrate TQM principles into their organization, because, ultimately, total quality management must have its foundation in understanding the health care consumer.

Eric N. Berkowitz
Professor and Head, Department of Marketing,
University of Massachusetts at Amherst
Editor, *Journal of Health Care Marketing*
President-Elect, Academy for Health Services Marketing

PREFACE

. . . .

I N 1986, Peter Francese and Brad Edmondson published a book entitled *Health Care Consumers*. Although it represented an important contribution to our understanding of health care consumer behavior, it was quickly dated. In fact, any work on health care consumers written since the mid-1980s is doomed to early obsolescence. Even works focusing on future developments in health behavior are quickly outdated in today's environment.

Developments of the 1980s permanently changed the nature of health care and set the stage for the trends of the 1990s. These changes included significant shifts in the settings for care and the types of practitioners used. They included the corporatization of health care providers in the form of large physician groups and hospital alliances, with health care organizations integrating both vertically and horizontally. This was followed by the corporatization of the purchasers of care, with insurers and other third-party payers negotiating services for their enrollees.

What accounts for the tremendous changes that health care has undergone? It is not the obvious answer—technology. In fact, the rapid change has occurred almost independent of medical clinical practice and research laboratory developments. The changes have been not so much in the treatment of disease, but in the structure, organization, functioning, and players of the health care system itself. The health care system has undergone a revolution in its mindset, totally redefining medical care (now health care) and reordering relationships that were thought to be carved in stone.

During the 1980s, patients came to be redefined as customers, medical procedures as products, and the community served as a market.

These factors, and particularly the emergence of the health care consumer, have ushered in the age of health care marketing. Of all the numerous changes that affected health care during the 1980s, this is probably the most significant. Changes in practice patterns, reimbursement procedures, and centers of power are not likely to have the impact that the emerging consumer orientation will.

Surprisingly little comprehensive treatment has been given to the topic of health care consumers in either academic or professional literature. Despite something of an explosion in the research completed during the last ten years on health care utilization patterns, little of this has been compiled into a definitive work. Hopefully, this book will fill some of the void in the literature, at least until the next series of changes.

Health Care Consumers in the 1990s is divided into nine chapters. It begins with an assessment of health care—and health care marketing—as the industry enters the 1990s. It ends with a prognosis for health care as the 20th century ends. In between, chapters two through eight review the nature of health care consumption (and health care consumers) and provide an overview of societal trends that will have an impact on health care consumption throughout the decade. Chapter four describes how the market for health services is segmented, and chapter five indicates ways to use this information to find prospective customers and transform them into loyal supporters of a health care organization.

Chapter six departs from the standard approach to health care consumers and focuses on the new "consumers" in the marketplace. These include physicians, insurers, alternative delivery systems, and the variety of other entities now serving as intermediaries between the health care provider and the patient. Chapters seven and eight are perhaps the most "technical" chapters. The former presents a practical review of the types of data needed for health care marketing—where to find them and how to use them. Chapter eight provides a straightforward assessment of various marketing techniques that might be employed in health care. An appendix provides more detailed guidance to sources of health care data.

RICHARD K. THOMAS
Memphis, Tennessee
April 1992

CHAPTER ONE

Health Care Enters the 1990s

W HO WOULD HAVE THOUGHT just a few years ago that most health care would be provided outside of hospitals; that "clerks" would be making decisions with regard to hospital admission, treatment, and discharge; that physicians would fall from their pedestals; that one of the major forces in health care would be our nation's large employers? Perhaps more important, who could have imagined the extent to which health care would become a business? Who would have thought that the nation's not-for-profit hospitals (some of which even have the word "charity" in their names) would adopt hard-nosed business principles in order to compete for patients?

Indeed, who could have foreseen the extent to which the "patient" would become a "customer?" When words like "consumer," "product," and "market" were introduced into health care during the 1980s, few observers anticipated that anyone would take them as seriously as they did. Agreed, these concepts provided a more practical way in which to view the components of the industry and provided a framework for business planning. But the industry has now gone further than anyone expected in acting as if patients (and physicians and employers) really are customers.

An emerging appreciation of the complexity of decision making about health care consumption has contributed to the obsolescence of our thinking (and our literature) on health care consumers. Conventional wisdom held that when people get sick they use health services. The only variation on that theme involved the notion that when doctors say people are sick (whether they are or not), they consume health services. Thus, in health care, the suppliers have paradoxically determined the demand for services.

In the 1980s, observers of health care were overwhelmed by the growing complexity of health behavior. Even prior to the formal introduction of marketing into health care, the industry implicitly took a mass market approach to its consumers. After all, everyone is susceptible to sickness, and health care is a product that everyone must consume at one time or another. As the results of market research became available, however, it quickly became clear that we had more misconceptions than insights about health care consumer behavior. Some of the findings were:

✔ The quality of care provided may not be as important to consumers as certain amenities.

✔ Consumers know even less about health care than was believed.

✔ There is wide variation in health behavior even among individuals with similar health problems.

✔ Women make most of the decisions about the use of health services.

✔ Consumers rely heavily on friends, relatives, and other nonmedical personnel in choosing a doctor or evaluating a hospital.

✔ Most health care consumers are poor "shoppers," since they are generally insulated from the cost of services.

Furthermore, despite the seeming universality of biological pathology, there is not one market for health care but many. Market research indicated that health care consumers, like consumers in other industries, are segmented by demographics, socioeconomic characteristics, lifestyles, and any number of other dimensions. Health care decision making is not simply the personal management of biological sickness by the individual, but a process involving his social and cultural milieu as well.

As if this did not complicate health care consumption enough, there are at least two other dimensions that further add to the complexity of this process. While demographics and other dimensions of market segmentation have been precisely linked to the demand for goods and services in a variety of industries, health care offers the added dimension of a linkage between health services need and segmentation factors. As it turns out, when it comes to health care, there is an imperfect relationship between the need for services and the demand for services. Many individuals who need health services do not consume them, while others with a limited need consume a large amount.

Another factor that confounds our understanding of the health care consumer relates to the existence of "third-party" entities that serve as an intermediary of sorts between the health care consumer and the point of sale. To a great extent, the decision to purchase is not made by the end user—the patient—but by a third party. Historically, this "gatekeeper" has been the phy-

HEALTH CARE

✔ *See Also*

For a visual depiction of the link between health services needs and wants, see page 91.

sician who officially declared the individual as "sick," ordered the tests, ordered hospitalization, prescribed drugs, and scheduled follow-up office visits. In a system that is physician-dominated, as ours has been, this is an important consideration. Convention held that the patient was to trust the doctor with his life, and this meant turning over most consumption decisions to this gatekeeper. More recently, the physician has been joined, and to a certain extent supplanted, by other decision makers. Third-party payers, such as insurance companies, managed-care programs, government health care financing agencies, and, increasingly, employers, have begun taking a more active role in decision making when it comes to health care consumption. Like the physician, these decision makers take the process out of the hands of the end user.

A final and related factor confounding the health care consumption process also relates to financing. The 1980s witnessed major changes in health care financing arrangements. Escalating costs and the cost-containment measures that resulted overrode virtually every other issue in health care. At the beginning of the 1980s, a variety of issues were the topic of professional meetings—manpower issues, quality issues, access issues. By mid-decade, every professional meeting, whether planned or not, appeared to focus on the financial aspects of the system.

The 1980s saw the introduction of strict cost-containment measures

Health Care Developments of the 1980s

THE 1980s will be remembered as a turning point for American health care. The developments of that decade transformed the industry and set the stage for trends that are shaping health care in the 1990s. The list below is not exhaustive but indicates some of the developments that have shaken the very foundation of the health care industry:

✔ *Introduction of competition.* Health care providers that had historically enjoyed essentially monopolistic or oligopolistic conditions suddenly found themselves facing cutthroat competition.

✔ *Shrinking market for hospital services.* Hospitals that had enjoyed unprecedented market growth for several decades suddenly found that the pie had stopped growing and, in many markets, had actually begun to shrink.

✔ *Major cost shifting and risk shifting.* Hospitals and physicians that had traditionally borne virtually no risk in providing services—their revenues were essentially guaranteed—found that those paying the bill wanted them to share some of the risk and suffer the consequences if there were cost "overruns."

✔ *Corporatization of buyers.* The "sellers" of health care who had enjoyed an effective monopoly in regard to supply suddenly found themselves facing entities that represented large groups of purchasers determined to extract favorable terms from suppliers.

✔ *Growing public dissatisfaction.* The public—including users, purchasers, and regulators of health services—became increasingly dissatisfied and demanded significant reforms on the part of hospitals and physicians previously considered beyond reproach.

▶

✔ *Major reductions in reimbursement.* In a development un-precedented in any other industry, health care providers faced changes in reimbursement procedures beyond their control that reduced their revenues so they received less payment for the same level of services.

✔ *Development of alternative sources of care.* Entrenched health services providers found that new organizations were eroding their market shares and capturing their customer bases by providing consumer-oriented services and elim-inating the high overhead associated with traditional care providers.

on the part of Medicare, the major component of government health spending. These were followed by similar attempts by other insurers to reduce spending. It was also the decade of the alternative-financing arrangement. Private insurers and employers who purchased the insur-ance introduced a variety of incentives to discourage inappropriate use of services. They raised deductibles, introduced copayment arrange-ments, and adjusted their premium schedules to encourage more judi-cious use of the health care system. They encouraged their enrollees to use outpatient settings and less expensive forms of treatment. Major employers attempted to cut out the middleman by becoming self in-sured.

Although health maintenance organizations (HMOs) had emerged in the 1970s, in the 1980s they began to replace much of the traditional indemnity insurance held by the population. Preferred provider organi-zations (PPOs) in their various guises also became common. This movement led to "managed care" as a major feature of the system. Managed-care programs attempted to control use of services by the in-sured or enrolled individual by "managing" the entire process from the prepatient stage through post-patient convalescence. These programs monitored the patient process every step of the way, using such mecha-nisms as preadmission screening, concurrent review of treatment, and discharge planning to assure that the patient did not receive inappropriate or unnecessary care.

In health care, the salesclerk's query, "How would you like to pay for that?" takes on new meaning. The standard insurance package, which covered most Americans not too many years ago, has become a dinosaur. A wide variety of traditional indemnity insurance packages now exists. These have been joined by the HMOs, PPOs, and a host of other managed-care arrangements. Add to these the government-sponsored programs such as CHAMPUS, Medicare, and Medicaid, and the financial complexity becomes mind-boggling. Furthermore, there is a growing population that must pay "out-of-pocket" due to a decline in employer-sponsored insurance coverage. This cash-on-the-barrelhead situation may appear attractive in view of the paperwork nightmare involved in the above-mentioned programs, but few people can actually pay for all of their health care needs.

The type and volume of health services consumed is mainly a function of the payment mechanism the patient has at his or her disposal. This means simply that two patients with similar health problems may consume different types and amounts of health services due to their differing coverage.

Shifting Power in Health Care

An important trend to develop out of this has been the shifting of decision making. Historically, decisions about the allocation of health care resources have been made by clinicians, primarily physicians. During the 1980s, conventional wisdom held that 70 percent to 80 percent of health care expenditures were the direct result of actions by physicians. A new force in health care emanating from the purchasers of care has resulted in a commensurate decline in the power of the physician. Changing consumer attitudes also reduced the physician's influence, and by the end of the 1980s, the physician's level of control had been reduced dramatically.

Many developments of the 1980s also served to push health care away from the hospital and into the outpatient arena. Technological advances, consumer preferences, and financial incentives combined to make outpatient care the treatment of choice. Patients who at one time would have gone nowhere but the hospital for urgent care, surgical procedures, diagnostic tests, and rehabilitation were now using outpatient facilities. Ambulatory-care services were much more in keeping with the changing mindset of the consumer, and nobody but the hospitals mourned the decline of inpatient care.

Redefining the Health Care Consumer

Perhaps the most significant development affecting health care marketing has been the redefining of the patient as consumer. The patient used to be something of a nonentity in the eyes of the health care providers. Patients routinely showed up and paid their bills. If a clinical issue had to be discussed, the physician would be consulted. If it had to do with the bill, it was the insurance company's responsibility. With limited decision-making power and limited financial input, the patient, especially the hospital patient, did not have much to do with the process but was dependent on the physician and the hospital.

By the mid-1980s, the decision-making powers of the patient began to be appreciated and, despite the development of corporate medicine, a majority of decisions regarding health care use are made by individuals. Well-educated consumers began asking tough questions and demanding participation in the treatment process. Consumers received more information about charges, procedures, qualifications, and insurance practices. They demanded that the system meet *their* needs, not the needs of physicians and hospital staff.

Hospitals, physicians, and other providers came to realize that an approach focusing on a one-time, ultra-dependent patient was not good for business in the long run. As these organizations became service-oriented, they began to shift the focus from the illness episode to the relationship. By the mid-1980s, in fact, hospitals were bringing in consultants from the hotel industry to help them understand and serve the needs of their consumers.

At the same time, a number of new "consumers" were identified in health care. Some actually were not so new, but they only recently have become recognized as customers. Hospitals came to see physicians as customers, physicians came to see other physicians as customers, man-aged-care providers came to see employers as customers, and so on. By 1990, the whole notion of the health care consumer had been revised, with significant implications for health care marketing.

Marketing and the Health Care Industry

During the 1980s, health care organizations (HCOs) began to realize that competition was here to stay. To succeed, they would have to oper-ate as businesses. They had to adopt practices long common in other industries. In particular, it required a shift from product orientation to service orientation. This shift gave impetus to the introduction of mar-keting into health care.

By the mid-1980s, marketing departments had sprung up in most HCOs. Just the other day, it seems, no hospital administrator would mention the word "marketing" above a whisper. Now, some even bear the title of vice president of marketing.

The introduction of marketing into health care and the subsequent relationship between the two has resembled a shaky romance. Health care organizations for the most part had no interest in marketing until the 1980s, and marketers saw no opportunities in health care until then. Once introduced, marketing and health care passed through a very ten-tative getting-to-know-you period. By the mid-1980s, however, it was a romance in full bloom with the two being seen everywhere together. HCOs were spending feverishly on their newfound consort, and mar-keters rushed to take advantage of the sudden burst of interest.

Unfortunately, HCOs did not see marketing for what it really was, having been taken in by the swaggering style of the promoter. They failed to do their market research homework, they rushed headlong into expensive media advertising, they took a mass marketing approach, they focused on image rather than programs, and they did not take steps to evaluate the effectiveness of their marketing activities. Thinking that advertising was marketing, health care administrators realized that they had been blinded by love. By the late 1980s, HCOs were slashing their marketing budgets, disbanding marketing staff, and gen-erally scaling back the relationship. Health care did not want to break it off altogether, but it did not want to continue spending on initiatives with vague benefits.

In a way, it was the worst possible situation for a marketer to step into. There was a tremendous sense of urgency that something had to be done by someone to address somebody's problems. Beyond this, few people had any idea of what marketing in health care was about or what a health care marketer was supposed to do. One thing was obvious: marketing health care was not like marketing any other product.

Both parties can probably be faulted for the shaky initial relationship. The marketers that health care imported from other industries added fuel to the fire by attempting to adapt techniques from banking, retailing, and other industries to health care. The first rule of marketing, of course, is to know your market, and they did not (actually, no one did). In effect, marketers were offering quick fixes and short-run answers in an industry that should be driven by long-term considerations. Even after some years on the job, few hospital marketers had developed a real marketing plan. They were too busy trying to explain health care to their ad agencies.

By the early 1990s, cooler heads prevailed. It was realized that marketing did not consist of spending truckloads of money on mass media. Progressive health care organizations began to pull back and assess their marketing objectives in a more reasonable light. They began to try to actually understand the market, their customers, and the motivations of consumers.

HEALTH CARE

✔ See Also

For a chart detailing the pros & cons of various forms of media advertising, see page 144.

Marketers, too, had learned some important lessons. Few marketing techniques could be transferred unmodified from other industries. The messages and the methods have to be tailored to health care. Sensitive issues are found here that are not a factor in other industries. Further, marketers are faced with the unique situation where the organization does not want to attract all potential customers, requiring a marketing selectivity unheard of in other industries.

In the 1990s, all parties are in a better position to rationally develop marketing programs. Health care marketers are beginning to understand the market and their customers. Some appreciation of what works

Who Needs Health Care Marketing?

PRIOR TO THE 1980s, marketing campaigns targeting health care consumers were relatively rare. This is not to say that certain segments of the health care industry were not heavily into marketing; some were. Noteworthy among these are pharmaceutical companies, whose spending on marketing is legendary. Their marketing efforts, however, targeted physicians as the key to distributing their products. Medical equipment and supply companies have also been heavily involved in marketing, but again, it has been aimed typically at health care organizations. Perhaps the insurance industry was the only one targeting consumers directly, with its advertising campaigns and legions of field representatives.

The 1980s witnessed two major departures from historical health care marketing patterns: targeting patients and the proliferation of both marketers and target audiences. By the mid-1980s, most care providers had realized it was a new world, and marketing was essential for organizational survival. Hospitals were most notable for their campaigns to woo patients to their facilities. Substance-abuse programs also became heavy marketers. Nursing homes, life-care centers, and other organizations followed. As "freestanding" facilities such as urgent- care centers, diagnostic centers, and ambulatory-surgery centers emerged, the intensity of marketing escalated. After all, these new forms of care had to carve out a niche from the existing market shares of established providers. They have been joined by home health agencies and other organizations that offer outreach-type care. Home infusion agencies, dialysis programs, and other facilities also joined the marketing parade.

Traditional indemnity insurers found that they were be-

▶

ing challenged by alternative forms of financing. Their historical approach to marketing was meek compared with campaigns launched by health maintenance organizations, preferred provider organizations, and other forms of "managed care." And these organizations have been joined by the growing number of organizations that provide related services either to providers such as hospitals or to the populations they serve. Organizations specializing in hospital financial analysis represent one category; those specializing in industrial health programs represent another. These entities have expanded the business-to-business marketing component of the industry.

Health care professionals have not escaped the marketing movement, either. While physicians have been slow to adopt some traditional media approaches to marketing, many have begun to advertise. They have also become more aggressive in marketing themselves to other physicians and negotiating arrangements with group purchasers of care. Dentists have followed a similar pattern. Certain other providers of care have been heavily involved in marketing for a decade. Many podiatrists, optometrists, and chiropractors are much less timid than physicians and dentists when it comes to traditional advertising. Even certain allied-health professionals have begun to market their programs, including psychologists and other counselors, physical therapists, and audiologists.

Who, then, needs health care marketing? In today's environment, every provider organization and health professional, all organizations that service providers, all organizations involved in the financing and processing of services—in short, anyone who interfaces with the health care industry needs marketing. For many, it is no longer a matter of market share, but a matter of survival.

and does not work is emerging. Some new techniques have been developed specifically for the health care market, there are now some legitimate health care marketers in the field, not just transplantees from other industries. This revived interest in marketing has come not a moment too soon. Every provider of health services, especially hospitals, realizes that in order to survive in an increasingly competitive environment, some type of marketing is necessary.

The health care industry has clearly been in a state of chaos, prompting a whole new set of questions on the part of health care providers. Who are the customers for a specific service? How can we position ourselves to appeal to the most "desirable" customers? How price-sensitive will the public be to a particular service? When is the right time to establish a satellite operation, and where should it be? In short, health care administrators began asking the kinds of questions that only a marketer could answer.

The Significance of the Individual Patient

In view of the various factors that influence health consumption decision making and, in many cases, actually "steer" the patient to one type of service or another, is it worthwhile to focus on the patient as consumer? To the extent that many choices are taken out of the hands of consumers, is it appropriate to target them at all?

In many ways, this is the best time in the history of health care to focus on the patient as a consumer. The developments of the 1980s have served to reduce the significance of hospital care, an area where the patient has had virtually no voice in the past. Someone else told him when to enter the hospital, what to do while he was there, and when to leave. Hospitals were organized to essentially eliminate any control or decision making on the part of the patient or his family.

One of the most important trends over the past decade has been the shift from inpatient care to outpatient care, expanding the role of the patient in decision making. There are a lot more choices for outpatient services than for inpatient services and fewer restrictions placed by third-party payers. Doctors are likely to choose their patients' hospital, but the patients themselves will choose the doctors, the fitness

From Medical Care to Health Care

DURING THE 1980s, the direction of the health care industry shifted away from "medical care" and toward "health care." Medical care is narrowly defined and refers primarily to those functions of the health care system under the influence of medical doctors. This concept encompasses the "clinical" aspects of care. Health care refers to any function that might be directly or indirectly related to preserving, maintaining, or enhancing health status. This concept includes formal activities such as visiting a physician or dentist, as well as informal activities such as preventive care, exercise, and proper diet.

The medical care orientation had its origins in turn-of-the-century scientific medicine. Medical scientists were, for the first time, able to diagnose and treat many of the conditions that accounted for much suffering and death among human populations. Linked inextricably to "germ theory," the medical model focused on specific disease organisms and their impact on human physiology, with medicine (here, drug therapy) the only appropriate response. Only legitimate physicians could diagnose and/or treat illnesses. The emergence of the medical model, thus, represented as much of a political victory for physicians as it did a scientific breakthrough.

Since the 1970s, however, there has been newfound understanding of the link between health status and lifestyle. Realizing that medical care has a limited ability to control the disorders of modern society prompted a move away from a strictly medical model of health and illness to a more social and psychological perspective.

The shift toward a health care orientation gained momentum during the 1980s. The shift in emphasis from

▶

acute illnesses to chronic illnesses further contributed to the devaluation of the medical model. A health care emphasis involves a much broader range of conditions than the medical care approach; many more aspects of care are important under the health care paradigm than under the traditional approach. Furthermore, important causal and treatment factors are quite different. It is one thing to link illness to the existence of a disease organization; it is much more complex to understand the part played by environment, lifestyles, and social stress in the onset and progression of disease.

Marketing medical care is one thing; marketing health care is quite another. The shift in orientation broadens the range of health problems and, as a result, the variety of treatment services. Furthermore, decisions related to medical care rest almost exclusively with the physician; under a health care orientation, a wider variety of participants become involved.

Marketing plays an important role in today's health care industry. As long as control is maintained by a select group of professionals, a real market does not exist. As the number of decision makers grows and the alternatives multiply, health care becomes more like other industries in its need for marketing.

---

programs they join, the diet programs they use, and the minor medical centers they visit. In fact, a recent study by National Research Corporation found that patients are now making more decisions about health care than at any time in the past.

Another important trend is the shift from medical care to health care. This shift effectively broadens the scope of health services consumption. Health care is no longer restricted to the use of formal services such as physicians and hospitals, but involves activities not previously considered related to medical care. These include services such as fitness programs, weight-reduction programs, counseling, lifestyle management, stress management, birthing classes, and a variety of other health services that do not necessarily involve hospitals and physicians.

These developments come at a time when consumers are becoming increasingly sensitive to both health care issues and health care costs. Growing segments of the market (and this includes the most desirable segments from a marketer's perspective) are paying increasing attention to their lifestyles and the way in which their behavior affects their health. At the same time, the population is becoming increasingly aware of health care costs as an issue. They are demanding more information on pricing, are willing to comparison shop, and are determined to get their money's worth. This doesn't necessarily mean that they will consume fewer health services because of the cost (they may, in fact, consume more), but that they want to use the "right" services at an appropriate price. If these decisions are left to physicians and hospitals, price is not likely to be a factor.

A final reason to retain a focus on the individual patient is the orientation of the dominant baby-boom generation. Boomers are not used to someone else making their decisions and are determined to see that their interests are addressed. The traditional doctor-patient relationship is the antithesis of the type of relationship this generation wants. Baby boomers want to participate in decision making, take an active role in their treatment, and otherwise control their own destinies.

The "New" Health Care

The U.S. began the 1980s with a health care system that had not changed much for several decades. True, Medicare and Medicaid were introduced during the 1960s, and these had an impact on the purchase of health care. For the most part, however, the basic structure of the system had not changed much. The typical consumer had a standard health-insurance package that was rubber-stamped by the insurer. The consumer had a regular physician whom he trusted and who was expected to provide guidance on the use of other health services. The hospital was the focal point for care and the technological imperative was widespread. Decisions were made the same way they had always been, the power rested in the same hands, and the same groups benefited and suffered as a result of the system.

By 1990, the health care system had been substantially transformed. The cost-containment measures introduced by Medicare had dramatically changed practice patterns. Traditional indemnity insurance had given way to various forms of managed-care programs. A large under-insured or uninsured population had developed. The traditional power-yielders and decision makers, the hospitals and physicians, had yielded control to third-party payers major care purchasers. The focal point of the risks had been altered just as dramatically as the power, with third-party payers, government insurance programs, and employers attempting to shift the risks to the hospital, the physician, or the patient.

These developments have permanently changed the character of the health care delivery system. Any one of these developments by itself would have shaken the industry, so it is no wonder that health care is still reeling from a decade that changed its world forever. Faced with overcapacity, declining utilization, and declining reimbursement for services, health care providers have been forced to compete for their share of a market that is shrinking in some ways. By the 1980s, the demand for traditional product offerings was becoming unpredictable, and the reimbursement environment was becoming increasingly uncertain. Hospitals were more affected by these developments than any other component of the system, and the level of hospital closures reached record levels. Physicians also were forced to modify their practice patterns. During the late 1980s, physicians experienced for the first time the leveling off (and in some cases actual declines) of patient visits and revenue.

HEALTH CARE

✔ HIGHLIGHT

In 1980, 73 hospitals closed. By 1988, that number had increased 45 percent, to 106.

After a decade of attempts, often extreme, to control costs and reduce health care expenditures, what is there to show for it? Nationally, health care costs continue to rise unabated, reaching for 12 percent of the gross national product and beyond. Those who are paying for care have on a sporadic basis experienced some improvement in their health

care burden. Overall, though, it appears that the demand for health services is insatiable; when utilization is reduced in one area, it increases
in another. A researcher for one of the major automakers has noted that
nearly a decade of major reorganizing of the company's health benefits
program toward a system that reduces utilization and saves money has
had virtually no affect on the upward trend of health care expenditures.

The dramatic changes in health care in the 1980s did not magically
end in 1990. In fact, the 1990s promise to be a decade of continued
transformation for health care. Some providers, especially physicians,
who escaped the 1980s relatively unscathed can expect to experience
the same pressure that hospitals felt in the last decade. New forms of
financing are expected to develop, and new organizational structures
are becoming common. Alliances that combine physicians and hospitals, hospitals and insurers, and a variety of other arrangements are
changing the structure of the industry.

CHAPTER TWO

....

Demographic Change and the Health Care Consumer

"By the turn of the century...new demographic patterns will be causing profound changes in health care. The trends will affect every sector of the health industry and every provider, insurer, and payer."

—Russell Coile, *health care futurist*

The New Demographic Order

America's health problems and health care system have been substantially shaped by demographic changes of the 20th century. The changing age structure of the population has resulted in an "epidemiological transition" that has dramatically altered the health problems that characterize American citizens. (*See page 20 for a discussion of the epidemiological transition.*) The nature of disease and the operation of the health care system have been altered as a result of changes in the nation's living standards, its educational level, and its lifestyles. These demographic changes have in fact overshadowed the much-publicized medical breakthroughs in their impact on the population's health status.

During this century, the U.S. has experienced unprecedented demographic change. While many of these changes have occurred in other industrialized nations as well, some have been unique to the U.S. The major demographic developments involved in this transition are outlined in the following sections.

Demography and the Health Care Consumer

Demographers think in terms of three major demographic processes. Fertility, mortality, and migration are important because they are the basic components of population change. To understand current and future demand for health services, one needs to understand these trends.

Change for a particular population is a function of fertility (persons added through birth), mortality (persons subtracted through death), and migration (persons either added or subtracted as a result of geographic mobility). The rate of "natural increase" for a population is a function of the difference between births and deaths. If births exceed deaths, a natural increase occurs. However, if deaths exceed births, a natural decrease occurs.

Fertility: the reproductive experience of a population.

Fertility analysis involves the study of the number and rate of births to a population, the characteristics of those giving birth, and the characteristics of the results (i.e., the offspring) of the fertility process. While the fertility process is not inherently linked to health care (e.g., some societies do not see childbirth as a medical process), the reproductive process has significant implications for health and health care in U.S. society. The level of fertility dictates the level of need for a variety of health-related services, including the number of hospitals in general and the number of obstetrical units in particular. The number of women who are pregnant at any point in time determines the need for ambulatory obstetric services. Pregnancy and associated physical conditions take up

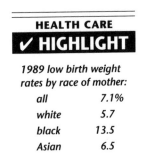

HEALTH CARE

✔ HIGHLIGHT

1989 low birth weight rates by race of mother:

all	*7.1%*
white	*5.7*
black	*13.5*
Asian	*6.5*
Hispanic	*6.2*

an increasing amount of outpatient clinic time, with prenatal and postnatal examinations becoming routine and pregnancy-related diagnostic tests becoming increasingly common. The demand for obstetrical services is complicated by the fact that fertility rates vary among various population segments. Some segments (e.g., relatively younger and older mothers) have above-average levels of medical complications.

The Epidemiological Transition

JUST AS industrializing nations underwent a demographic transition during the 19th century, "mature" industrial nations such as the United States experienced an *epidemiological transition* during the 20th century. Driven by the changing age structure of U.S. society, the epidemiological transition involved the diminution of acute health conditions and the emergence of chronic health conditions as the focal point of the health care system. At the beginning of this century, acute conditions were the most common health problems and the leading killers. Today, chronic conditions account for the lion's share of health problems and deaths.

Acute conditions involve problems that might be considered "episodic" or involve a one-time occurrence. Acute conditions are characterized by fairly direct causation (e.g., exposure to a disease organism or an accident), relatively rapid onset, rapid progression and short duration, and a disposition involving either recovery or death. From an epidemiological perspective, the entire population is generally at risk from acute conditions, since they are no respecters of age, sex, race, or social class. Colds, infectious diseases, and injuries are typical acute conditions.

Chronic conditions are characterized by a relatively complex etiology, slow onset and progression, and no clear-cut disposition. Unlike many acute conditions, most chronic conditions are not self-limiting nor do they result directly in death. Also, chronic conditions typically cannot be cured, only managed. Unlike acute conditions, chronic conditions (due to their link with nonbiological factors) tend to be distributed unevenly within a population, reflecting differences in socioeconomic conditions, lifestyles, and environmental factors. Examples of chronic conditions include hypertension, diabetes, arthritis, and chronic obstructive respiratory disease.

Twentieth-century America has become increasingly dominated by chronic conditions. They have replaced acute condi-

▶

tions as the major causes of morbidity, disability, and mortality. This shift has been problematic for American medicine, which had emphasized treatment and cure but not disease management. Developments in medical education, biomedical research, and insurance coverage have not kept pace with this shift from acute to chronic conditions.

Once chronic conditions become predominant, the composition of the population becomes a powerful predictor of both health status and health behavior, because chronic conditions can sometimes be linked closely to lifestyle. Here, demographic and socioeconomic information becomes key to understanding the nature of health and illness in society.

To develop health care marketing, one must appreciate these issues. If the most common health problems are acute conditions, there is a reasonably close correlation between health problems and health services utilization. Acute conditions typically require "one-shot" medical responses—administering antibiotics, setting a fracture, removing an appendix.

The situation is quite different with chronic conditions. For one thing, as mentioned above, chronic conditions tend to be more segmented within the population than are acute conditions. Also, since chronic conditions do not usually constitute immediate life-or-death situations, there is more room for decision making on the part of the patient or his family. The notion of "elective" surgery, in fact, is a product of the epidemiological transition.

This shift, of course, has significant implications for health care marketing. When most health problems are emergencies, there is not much room for the marketer. However, if the dominant conditions are arthritis, hypertension, obesity, and neurosis, the patient becomes a consumer. As a consumer, she makes choices about physicians, medications, and forms of treatment. Witness the market that has developed almost overnight for cholesterol-reducing drugs. As chronic conditions begin to dominate, individuals have come to play a larger role in their own health care. These individuals then become targets for marketers who want to influence their health care consumption decisions.

Mortality: the level of death characterizing a population.

Mortality analysis studies the relationship between the number and rate of deaths and the size and characteristics of the population. As with fertility, there are wide variations in death rates among various segments of the population. The mortality pattern of a society has significant implications for the health care system, and it shapes the demand for medical care, drugs and supplies, health care facilities, and health manpower.

Perhaps more important than the level of mortality is a population's cause-of-death configuration. Cause of death reflects the health problems that characterize a society and determines the types of services required. When diseases (e.g., small pox) are eliminated as major causes of death, the market for care related to those diseases is reduced. As other conditions (e.g., AIDS) surface as major killers, the market for services related to these conditions expands. Not only does the cause of death dictate the level and types of health services used (many people consume more health services during their last month than during the entire rest of their lives), it determines the type and extent of "death prevention" programs. Clearly, efforts to reduce deaths from lung cancer and heart disease have spawned a number of industries for health-related services.

Migration: the movement of individuals and groups from one geographic area to another.

While fertility and mortality are clear-cut, easily measured events, migration is more problematic. It may involve a series of moves, return migration, and repeat migration. Migration can be temporary or permanent, voluntary or involuntary.

Demographers divide migration into two major categories: internal migration and international migration. Internal migration refers to movement *within* a particular country or other area. There is no systematic way to track internal migration in the U.S. International migration is movement from one country to another. In the U.S., the Immigration and Naturalization Service maintains fairly accurate records on legal immigration. On the other hand, much illegal immigration is undocumented, and emigration from the U.S. is not well documented.

The importance of migration in relation to the demand for health services cannot be overemphasized. Immigrants to the U.S. have often introduced new diseases or reintroduced old ones. And in a relatively short period of time, the population of a health service area can experience tremendous growth or loss or a significant change in its composition due to migration, which in turn can create extreme mismatches between the population and the health services available.

Population Growth

Throughout the 20th century, the U.S. population has been characterized by steady and sometimes substantial growth. Although slow-growing relative to many of the world's developing countries, population growth assured a steady increase in the supply of health care consumers. In fact, from World War II through the 1980s, population growth exceeded the increase in the supply of physicians and many other types of health services.

Over recent decades, however, U.S. population growth has been slowing in both numbers and percentages. The 1980s experienced the slowest growth rate since the Depression, at less than 1 percent per year. Nevertheless, this rate exceeds those of Europe and Japan, which grew by 3 percent and 6 percent, respectively, during the 1980s. The striking thing about this is that one-third of U.S. population growth was accounted for by immigration, much of it from Asia.

Despite slowing population growth, substantial numbers are still being added to the U.S. population. However, the population increase between 1990 and 2000 is expected to be less than 18 million. This compares with numerical increases of more than 23 million for each of the previous five decades. As the baby boomlet of the early 1990s subsides, immigration will account for an even greater share of population growth. "Natural increase"—the excess of births over deaths—will account for a declining share. This shift in the components of growth has obvious implications for health services demand. Additions to the population by virtue of birth have quite different health care needs than do additions to the population via immigration.

It is important to note that most health care markets are *local* markets and, as such, are less impacted by national population trends than by regional and local trends. There is considerable variation in patterns of population growth and decline from community to community and from market to market. Thus, population change in each health care service area must be examined in its own right.

Population Composition

Age Distribution.   The most significant demographic development in the U.S. during this century has been the restructuring of the population's age distribution. The demographic transition (i.e., the stabilizing of birth rates and death rates at relatively low levels) was more or less completed early in the century. Since then, the American population has undergone a long and steady process of aging. The combined effects of decreasing mortality, mid-century declines in immigration, and long-term decline in fertility have resulted in a population that is becoming older decade by decade. With each passing year, the

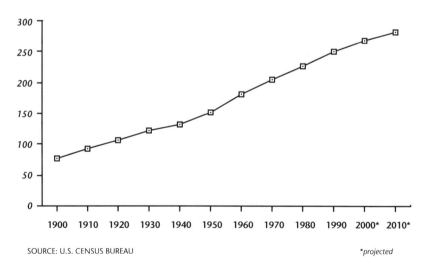

✔ *U.S. Population Growth Trends*

population in millions

SOURCE: U.S. CENSUS BUREAU   *projected*

American population sets a new record for median age. During the 1990s, the median age will increase from 33 to 36 years. The bulk of the population is now concentrated in the 30-plus age cohorts, with no net growth expected for the under-45 population during the 1990s. Any population increases recorded will be among the 45-plus population. This trend cannot be expected to diminish until well into the 21st century. As Barbara Everitt Bryant, director of the United States Census Bureau, notes: "We have never been this old before, and we will never be this young again. . . ."

As the population ages, numerous effects on the demand for health services are introduced. Older populations in general require more health services than do younger populations, especially hospital care and more intensive services. Thus, as the population pyramid becomes more "mature," the demand for health services increases proportionately. The elderly (aged 65 or older) currently account for 12 percent of the population and 31 percent of hospital admissions, where they stay longer and accumulate more expenses per admission than the nonelderly. Similarly, the elderly account for 40 percent to 50 percent of physician office visits. The elderly not only need more care, but they need *different* care. U.S. society faces the challenge of developing a new spectrum of services for a population that has never existed before. Already life-care communities and elder-care programs are becoming common.

The huge baby-boom generation is now entering its late 40s. Although the health conditions of aging begin to accumulate after age 45, the age at which the demand for health services escalates has steadily risen. Today, most people remain relatively healthy through their 60s. This means that it will be another 20 years before the heaviest pressure will be felt within the health care system.

Perhaps more important than any increase in overall demand for health services is the shift in demand by type of service. In fact, it is argued that older people, up to a point at least, do not have more health problems than younger people; they simply have different ones. A young population is characterized by a high level of acute conditions, conditions that tend to be short-lived and are easily treated. An older population is characterized by chronic conditions that are of long duration and essentially incurable, but only manageable. In the 1990s, chronic health conditions have replaced acute conditions as the most common problems and leading killers of the population.

The other significant implication of the changing age structure is the uneven distribution of population among the various age categeories. The population pyramids below and at right show unprecedented differences in the sizes of various age groups. Some of the differences in the size of adjacent categories are quite dramatic. The major factor accounting for these irregularities, of course, is the existence of the dominant baby-boom generation. It is considerably larger than the cohorts

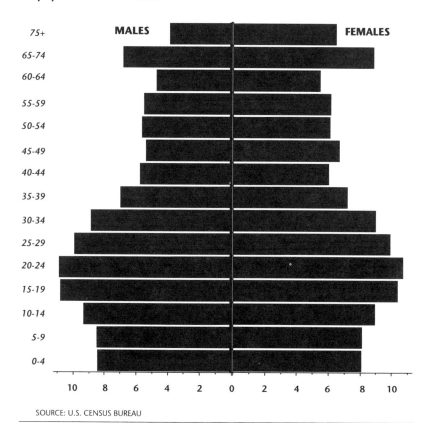

✔ U.S. Age Pyramid 1980

population in millions

SOURCE: U.S. CENSUS BUREAU

preceding it or following it. Furthermore, the baby boomlet of the 1980s and early 1990s is creating another, albeit less dramatic, irregularity in the age structure.

The operation of many institutions depends on the orderly flow of population from category to category. Obvious examples involve education and the economy. In the case of the latter, we see periods of labor surpluses alternating with periods of labor shortages. In addition, programs like Social Security rely on a steady stream of new workers entering at the bottom of the population pyramid to "support" the older age groups. In health care, the implications are most obvious in the

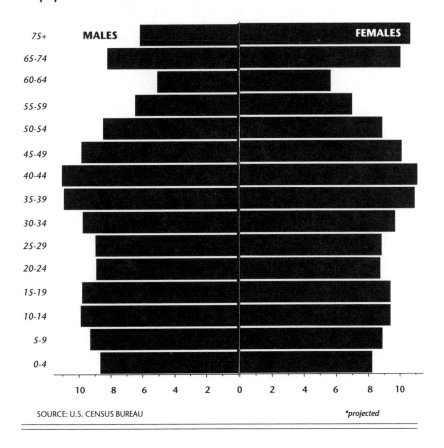

✔ **U.S. Age Pyramid 2000***

population in millions

SOURCE: U.S. CENSUS BUREAU   *projected*

✔ Age Time Trends

population in millions

YOUTH AGED 0 TO 14

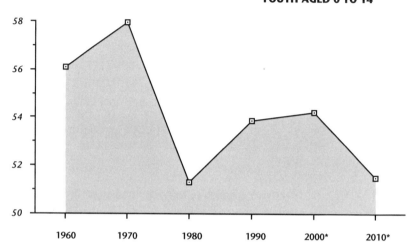

YOUTH AGED 15 TO 24

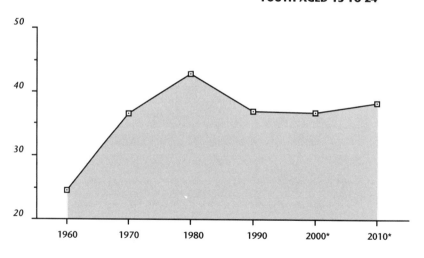

SOURCE: U.S. CENSUS BUREAU　　　　　　　　　　*projected

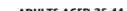

✔ Age Time Trends

population in millions

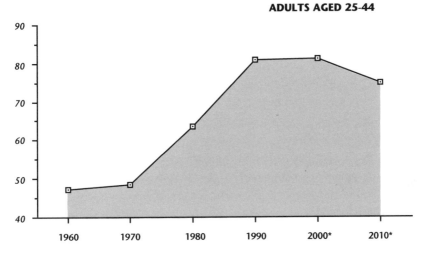

ADULTS AGED 25-44

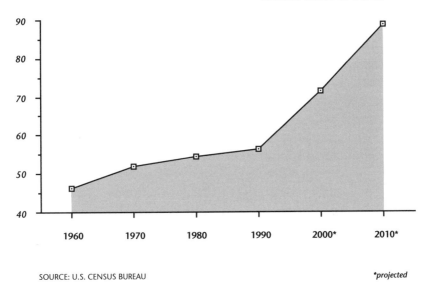

ADULTS AGED 45 TO 64

SOURCE: U.S. CENSUS BUREAU   *projected*

✔ Age Time Trends: The Elderly

population in millions

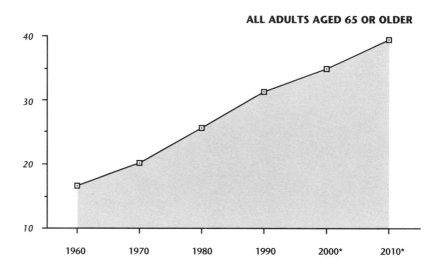

ALL ADULTS AGED 65 OR OLDER

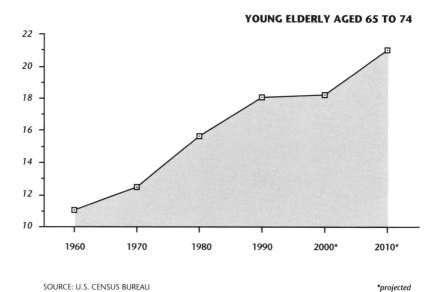

YOUNG ELDERLY AGED 65 TO 74

SOURCE: U.S. CENSUS BUREAU   *projected*

✔ *Age Time Trends: The Elderly*

population in millions

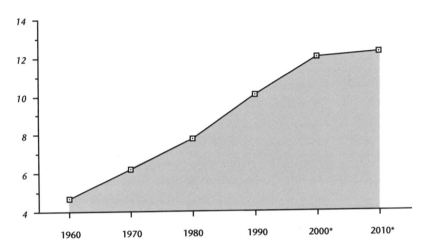

ELDERLY AGED 75 TO 84

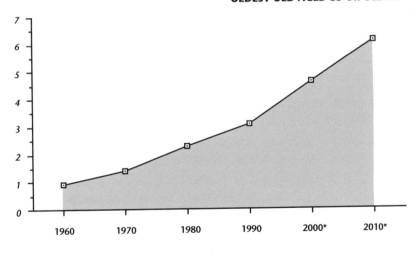

OLDEST OLD AGED 85 OR OLDER

SOURCE: U.S. CENSUS BUREAU   **projected*

funding of Medicare. In view of the changing age structure, the demand for Medicare services will soon exceed the ability of the system to pay for them.

Sex Distribution.   The developments of this century have served to modify the population's sex distribution along with its age structure. Historically, populations have contained a slightly higher proportion of males than females. More boys are born than girls, and relatively young populations tend to be numerically dominated by males. The significant reduction in maternal mortality occurring early in this century helped reduce some of the male/female differential. Today, however, the major factor is the aging of the population. Because men live an average of seven years less than women, as a population ages it becomes more female dominated. By the young-adult years, females begin to dominate numerically, and by the time they reach the oldest age cohorts, there are several times as many women as men.

The significance of the "feminization" of American society cannot be overstated. The numerical increase per se is not as important as the changes that have accompanied it. Today, for example, more than 25 million women now head their own households. Women account for 60 percent of single-person households and 86 percent of single-parent households.

These facts are particularly significant for health care. Women tend to be the major decision makers with regard to health care consumption in U.S. society. The unprecedented independence they have achieved has changed the ground rules for health care marketing. Even more important, women use health services much more frequently than men. They are sick more often, go to the doctor more often, and use more related services such as emotional counseling and weight-loss programs. In fact, at two key points in the lifecycle—during the childbearing years and the senior years—the overwhelming majority of health services are utilized by women. As the population continues to age, the health care system will become more and more female dominated. Not only do women have different needs, but they must be approached in a different manner than men. The fact that most women today work outside the home adds an additional dimension to their situation. With their growing independence, they have different expectations and will demand a system that is sensitive to their needs.

Racial and Ethnic Diversity.   The 1980s was a decade of increasing racial and ethnic diversity in the U.S. Although blacks, Hispanics, and Asians are still minorities, their numbers and influence are growing faster than those of non-Hispanic whites. In fact, non-Hispanic whites became a minority of the population in some U.S. cities during the 1980s. By the end of the 1990s, the state of California is expected to record a "minority majority," with Texas and Florida not too far behind.

During the 1980s, the black population grew nearly one-and-a-half times faster than the population overall. Blacks now comprise 12 percent of the U.S. population. This growth has been spurred by the higher fertility rates of the black population. As a result, this segment of the population contains higher proportions of children and lower proportions of the elderly than the total population.

The Asian population more than doubled in number during the 1980s, growing from 3.5 million to more than 7 million. In 1990, it made up 3 percent of the total U.S. population. Much of this group's growth is from immigration. Asian influence within American society

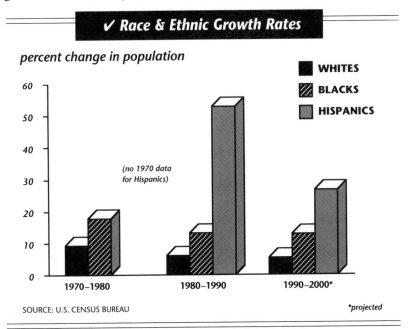

✔ *Race & Ethnic Growth Rates*

percent change in population

SOURCE: U.S. CENSUS BUREAU   *projected*

is growing at least as fast as the population, since Asian Americans tend to be even more affluent than majority non-Hispanic whites.

The Hispanic population grew 53 percent during the 1980s and now accounts for 9 percent of the population. The Asian and Hispanic populations are both increasing much faster than the black population, due to the combined effects of immigration and fertility. As in the case of the black population, however, these growth rates suggest a younger age structure than that of the nation as a whole. When all of these trends are considered, the bottom line is: one-fourth of U.S. residents are blacks, Hispanics, Asians or Pacific Islanders, American Indians, Eskimos, or Aleuts. Even more striking is the fact that nearly half—48 percent—of the nation's children in 1990 were racial or ethnic minorities. From a marketer's perspective, this suggests, among other things, that ethnic markets are family markets.

The ethnic market itself is diverse. Grouping the ethnic population into broad categories such as Hispanic or Asian masks a lot of the diversity reflected in geographic and subcultural differences. Historically, Europeans dominated the makeup of immigrant populations entering the U.S. At the turn of the century, Europeans accounted for more than 90 percent of all immigrants; by the late 1980s, they comprised only about 10 percent. On the other hand, Asians, who accounted for only 6 percent of immigrants as recently as the 1950s, comprised nearly half by 1990. Similarly, immigrants from other countries in the Western Hemisphere (mostly Latin Americans) increased their share from less than 5 percent in the early 1900s to about 40 percent in 1990. In 1950, the number of African immigrants was negligible; by the late 1980s, they accounted for 3 percent of all immigrants.

The Immigration Act of 1990 not only assures a steady flow of immigrants into the U.S. but actually has the intent of increasing the diversity of the immigrant pool. From a health care perspective, these new immigrants are quite different from the stereotyped European immigrant who shares many of the norms and values of middle America. New Americans from Vietnam, Ethiopia, the former Soviet Union, Lebanon, Haiti, and Mexico represent diverse cultures, all of which are significantly different from what is thought of as "American." They have different attitudes toward the health care system, they represent different patterns of health behavior, and they bring with them a different set of health problems.

Socioeconomic Characteristics

In many ways, the most significant demographic changes that have occurred relate to family and household structure, especially in the implications they have for the level of health problems, the amount of services used, and the ability to pay for health care.

Marital Status.   Since the family-building period of the 1950s and 1960s, revolutionary changes have occurred in marital status. Americans traditionally have been noteworthy for their rate of marriage. For most of this nation's history, virtually everyone (more than 95 percent) eventually married, at a rate effectively surpassing those of most other societies. From the 1970s on, however, several trends have changed this. Americans delayed marriage to a later age, and a growing number decided not to marry at all. By 1990, the ever-married rate of 95 percent had dropped to 91 percent for women and 88 percent for men. Not only were there fewer marriages, but a growing proportion of married couples were opting to have fewer children or none at all.

Decreased marriage rates have resulted in changes in the proportions in other marital statuses. The proportion of the population that is divorced has continued to increase, and the proportion that has never married has reached record levels. As a result of the aging of the population, the proportion widowed has also reached historic highs. Individuals in different marital statuses differ in both health status and health services use. Changes in the proportion single, married, divorced, and widowed will result in changes in the level and nature of health problems and in the demand for various health services.

Family and Household Structure.   Trends in individual marital status are reflected in the changing structure of American families and households. "Family" refers to a group of related individuals living under the same roof. "Household" refers to one or more individuals living together whether or not they are related. There are important differences between the two.

One of the most significant consequences of the 1990 census has been the documentation of the gradual demise of the traditional American family. In fact, there appears to no longer be a "typical" American family, at least in the sense of a numerical majority. As shown in the following table, by 1990 the most common type of family was the married couple without children under age 18. This family type accounted for 29 percent of all households. They are followed by married couples with children (26 percent) and single-parent families (15 percent). Each of these family types obviously has different needs and behaves differently with regard to health care consumption.

The most notable characteristic of American households in the late 20th century is the number of people living alone. Once a rarity, they now account for one in six households. The number of single-person households is growing so fast, in fact, that this trend alone promises to place inordinate pressure on the nation's housing stock.

These changes in family and household structure have important implications for health care. Individuals who are married or are living in some sort of satisfactory household arrangement tend to have fewer health problems and make better use of the health care system. They

✔ Household Type

	1960	1970	1980	1990
FAMILIES	**85.0%**	**81.2%**	**73.7%**	**70.8%**
Married couple	74.3	70.5	60.8	56.0
with children under age 18	44.3	40.3	30.9	26.3
Female-headed	8.4	8.7	10.8	11.7
with children under age 18	4.0	4.5	6.7	7.1
Male-headed	2.3	1.9	2.1	3.1
NONFAMILIES	**15.0%**	**18.8%**	**26.3%**	**29.2%**
Living alone	13.1	17.1	22.7	24.6
Living with nonrelatives	1.9	1.7	3.6	4.6

SOURCE: CURRENT POPULATION SURVEYS, U.S. CENSUS BUREAU

tend to have healthier lifestyles and benefit from the availability of health-promoting social support. In contrast, individuals who are divorced, single, widowed, or otherwise on their own suffer more from both physical and mental disorders. They report more illness symptoms, they suffer more serious conditions, and they have higher mortality rates. They are less likely to receive appropriate medical care. Furthermore, they are less likely to be adequately insured than the traditional married-couple household.

Educational Level. The U.S. population of the 20th century has been characterized by an increasing education level. Americans have become the best-educated population in the world. Despite this, there are large segments of the population whose educational levels fall below minimal standards established in other countries. As with income, there appears to be a widening gap between the well educated and the poorly educated in U.S. society.

The types of health problems that exist correlate with educational level, as does the use of services. Better-educated populations tend to be healthier and ostensibly require fewer health services. Yet the better educated are more sensitive to the benefits of health services; not only do they receive more frequent routine medical and dental care, they use more preventive services such as prenatal care. From a marketer's perspective, a better-educated consumer population has a better understanding of health issues, thereby requiring more sophisticated marketing approaches.

Occupational/Industrial Distribution. During this century, the American economy has shifted from agrarian to industrial to service. The type of economy influences the kinds of health problems that exist and thus the level of demand for certain services. The nature of the economic system also determines the society's ability to pay, particularly as it relates to the availability of employer-sponsored health insurance. Many observers also contend that the overall standard of living has risen, which has been a major factor in improving the health status of the population and extending life expectancy.

Income Distribution. During the 20th century, significant redistribution of income has occurred. Much of the century was characterized

The Dual Market for Health Care

THE MARKET for health care was once considered homogeneous and undifferentiated. Consumers were similar, each with a regular physician and a standardized way of paying for health care, and a mass marketing approach was considered adequate for targeting this market. Today, the health care market is highly segmented, classified by age, sex, lifestyle, and ability to pay. Many segment-oriented services (e.g., women's care and geriatric care) have developed. By the late 1980s, target marketing became common as health care marketers attempted to match services and messages with various market segments.

While health care marketers have been struggling with the intricacies of market segmentation, it appears that a dual health care market has been emerging. There seems to be a significant split based on age that divides an older "traditional" market from a youthful "modern" one. Roughly speaking, the cut divides those born before and after World War II, or people currently aged 45 or older from those under age 45. This rift in the health care market appears strong enough to override other dimensions of segmentation.

"Traditional" health care consumers are characterized by attitudes and values formed during the Depression and World War II. The uncertainties of those times created a generation that embraces security, conformity, and authority. It favors a traditional approach to health problems, with its emphasis on technology, treatment, and cure. Traditionalists encourage the health care system to manage them medically and tend to abdicate responsibility for their own health.

Traditional consumers believe cost is not a consideration when it comes to care. They have established relationships with doctors and experience with specific hospitals. The physician is their primary source of information. Traditional health care con-

▶

sumers are likely to be covered by standard health insurance policies. These characteristics make for a "good patient" in the eyes of physicians and hospital administrators. This patient respects the system, supports its basic values, follows the doctor's orders, and pays the bill.

Modern health care consumers have emerged from a different context than their parents. They were born into a world of comparative stability and unprecedented affluence. This generation is averse to turning control over to the health care system or any other formal organization. Unlike their elders, members of this group are skeptical about the benefits of physician care and hospitalization. This attitude, coupled with their better health, means that they have little experience with doctors, hospitals, and other health services, and are less likely than older consumers to have a doctor. They recognize the shortcomings of a system that emphasizes care for the sick, not prevention of sickness.

Modern health care consumers are causing a dramatic shift in health care settings. They shun the more formalized inpatient setting in favor of speedier outpatient care with its convenience and lower cost. Those under age 45 are the primary customers of minor emergency centers, surgicenters, and other freestanding clinics. The modern consumer has led the movement away from traditional health insurance; membership in alternative financing programs is dominated by people under age 45.

Health care marketers need to recognize that a dual health care market exists. Traditional consumers will continue to demand specialized inpatient services, and they will be willing to pay the price. Modern consumers want outpatient care, convenience, speed, and low cost. They also want to play a role in the therapeutic process.

A dual health care market complicates product mix and service delivery for health care providers. Focusing on either traditionals or moderns may unnecessarily limit the customer base, yet it may be difficult to develop a service mix that appeals to both groups. Clearly, these two groups require distinct

▶

marketing approaches.

As modern consumers age, can they be expected to become more traditional? While it is true that past generations tended to become like their parents as they got older, this is not likely to be the case with the modern health care consumer. The characteristics of moderns are firmly rooted in their postwar experiences, experiences that set them apart from their predecessors. Consequently, the dual health care market will eventually be replaced by the modern market. Health care marketers must monitor these changes if they expect to succeed in today's, and tomorrow's, health care environment.

by a "democratization" of wealth in the U.S. Incomes have steadily risen for decades, and the rise of a dominant middle class has been a hallmark of the U.S. economy. By the end of the 1980s, however, there was evidence of a widening gap in income distribution. The gap between the poorest segments and the most affluent segments appears to be increasing again. Since income is one of the best predictors of both health status and health services use, a change of this type will have important implications for the health care system.

Lifestyle Trends

This century has witnessed a lifestyle revolution in the U.S. Two decades ago, futurists were predicting the elimination of lifestyle differences as the mass media encouraged the standardization of the American way of life. By the 1980s, it was clear that this homogenization was not going to occur; if anything, lifestyle differences were being augmented. Regional differences remained strong, and the influx of new and culturally different immigrants further added to the heterogeneity of U.S. society.

While some lifestyle differences are a function of demographic differences, many lifestyles cross demographic lines. One of the surprises for marketers in the 1980s was the realization that demographically similar groups may vary significantly in lifestyle. Population segments that are similar in age and income, for example, may vary considerably in attitudes, values, and consumer behavior patterns.

As a society, Americans have been reevaluating many values that relate to health care. We have come to consider health care as a right but at the same time have become more realistic about our ability to pay for it. Many have become somewhat disenchanted with technology and, in terms of health care, are looking for a little less high tech and a little more high touch. Baby boomers do not have the same confidence in the institutions that their forefathers naïvely accepted; they are skeptical of hospitals, physicians, and insurance companies. They are used to charting their own courses, and the dependence that the health care system has historically demanded of patients does not sit well with this group. They want to be involved, participate in the process, and have ultimate say over what happens to them.

The "Fracturing" of American Society

Futurists of the 1960s and 1970s repeatedly predicted the effective homogenization of U.S. society by the year 2000, if not sooner. They foresaw rapid movement toward a common dialect, culture, and lifestyle under the inescapable influence of the mass media and social conformity. They were convinced that by the end of the century, everyone would speak with a midwestern accent and be characterized by uniform styles of dress, diet, and recreational activities.

If anything, the turn of the century will witness an American population more heterogeneous than it has been in generations. Despite unprecedented interregional mobility, regional differences have not only persisted but appear to have become more entrenched. New waves of immigrants have led to a reemergence of ethnic America, but this time the newcomers are from different cultures than previous immigrants, and to a certain extent, resist assimilation.

Ample evidence indicates that U.S. society is undergoing something of a "fracturing" process. Much of this trend has its roots in demographic processes, including the consequences of fertility and mortality over the past several decades. Demographically, today's population is characterized by irregularity in age cohorts—the huge baby-boom cohort is much larger than the cohorts before and after. Changes in family structure and in age distribution have resulted in a variety of new population segments, including a large older unmarried category, a post-marital category, an empty-nest category, and so forth.

The fracturing of U.S. society can be seen in other ways as well. There seems to be a rift occurring in educational attainment between the college-educated and the noncollege-educated. It seems that we are becoming a nation of Ph.D.s and functional illiterates with little in between. This has resulted in a dual labor market of highly skilled and less skilled workers. This in turn is causing a more polarized income distribution. After decades of convergence, we are becoming once again a nation of haves and have-nots.

There also appears to be fracturing along a variety of social and cultural dimensions. In addition to the growing ethnic diversity and persistent regionalism noted above, America has witnessed an emergence of different lifestyles related to different sexual preferences and religious affiliations.

These emerging segments of the population, whether new immigrants, single parents, or those with gay lifestyles, will have diverse health problems and health service needs. They will complicate an already complex market. Marketers must go well beyond traditional demographic targeting in order to appreciate and capitalize on the diverse interests of many societal segments.

Demographic Change in the 1990s

Most demographic trends of the 1990s are well underway, and it is possible to chart their course throughout the decade. It is clear that the U.S. population will continue to age. Baby boomers are moving through their 30s and 40s, and the life expectancy of those already old by yesterday's standards will be lengthened even more. Despite the current baby boomlet, additions of youth to the population cannot compete with the juggernaut of aging. In fact, if it were not for the current high levels of immigration, the population would be aging even faster.

The aging of the population has resulted in a need to differentiate among the oldest age cohorts. The distinction between the young-old, the middle-old, and the old-old will become even clearer. Perhaps this distinction is no clearer anywhere than with health care. There are major differences between the active 60s, the declining 70s, and the frail 80s. The young-old of today are similar to the 55-year-olds of the past, requiring management of chronic conditions. The middle-old begin to experience greater need for intensive services, especially hospital care. The old-old epitomize the stereotypical elderly of the past, with many suffering from severe disabilities and/or being restricted to institutions.

The ethnic and racial diversification of American society will also continue. Immigration from will ensure the addition of new Americans with diverse cultural backgrounds. Furthermore, some observers contend that the melting pot process is not operating as in the past. These new immigrants are not assimilating into American society in the same manner as their predecessors, and we are moving toward a pluralistic society composed of a variety of culturally different segments.

HEALTH CARE

✔ INSIGHT

New consumer segments will demand innovation from health care providers.

The 1990s will also witness the continued diversification of household types. The changes of the 1980s have required a redefinition of "family" and "household." The traditional notion of life cycles has lost its usefulness as a model for predicting consumption, as more and more individuals violate the traditional life-cycle progression.

Many of these changes will contribute to the further development of new demographic categories. The 1980s engendered the emergence of a post-marital segment, a never-married segment, a single-parent segment, a professional woman segment, and so forth. The 1990s will continue to witness groundbreaking developments in the creation of new demographic categories. The health care needs of these new categories will set them apart from traditional societal segments and will call for innovations on the part of those who seek to serve their health care needs.

Population redistribution will continue in the 1990s, but probably not at the rate of previous decades. Growth will continue to be faster in the South and West, but the level of mobility of the U.S. population is decreasing. In other words, people are moving less. The major region-to-region shifts of the past are not expected to continue at the same level as the rate of internal migration slows.

Not only are ethnic and national differences being preserved and emphasized, regional differences remain strong. There also appears to be a divergence of income, education, and lifestyle. For marketers, these trends contribute to the segmentation of the market and make stereotyping of consumer groups almost impossible.

The U.S. population of 2000 will be different from that of 1990. It will not only be different demographically, but its health needs, its use patterns, and its perceptions of the health care system will be different. Those who have an interest in the health care consumer must be prepared to address the changes engendered by these trends.

Implications for the Health Care Consumer

The health care consumer is undergoing considerable transformation. Once considered a nonentity who really did not play a part in the health care system, by both the system and the consumer herself, the end user of health services is now seen in a new light. It may not be so much that the individual health care consumer is changing but that the overall consumer market is changed by demographic shifts.

For decades, the typical consumption unit for health services has been the traditional American family, with mother and father, a couple of children, and standard health insurance. Decisions were typically made by an adult member of the household and usually by the husband and wife jointly. The typical consumer was a young white adult, confident in the health care system. He had a moderate level of education, enough to make him aware of the importance of health services but not enough to make him think he knew anything about medicine.

Today's health care consumer—and the pattern for the 1990s—is essentially "none of the above." The consumption unit may be a household with husband, wife, and children, but it is just as likely to be a single mother, a cohabiting couple, or an elderly widow living alone. The health care decision maker is increasingly likely to be female. And the decision maker now is less likely to be a non-Hispanic white than in the past. While consumers are better educated overall, there is no standard level of education. If current trends continue, we can predict a divergence of educational levels; patients will either be highly educated or close to functionally illiterate. Those who are well educated will know a lot about health care and will want to participate in the   process.

The health care consumer is also being changed by socioeconomic trends. Since World War II, it has been assumed that the typical consumer is middle class, with all that implies for consumption patterns. The middle class will remain important in the 1990s. However, averages are misleading. If income distribution trends continue, the health care consumer can expect to be either relatively affluent or relatively poor, with a decreasing common ground in between. Given the importance of insurance coverage in the financing of health care, this shift is of considerable significance.

The 1980s witnessed an unprecedented increase in the number of medically uninsured Americans. By the end of the decade, the number of individuals lacking health insurance was placed in the 35 million range, with some estimates exceeding 37 million. This does not include the additional millions who are underinsured or those who are only marginally covered by the Medicaid program. Unfortunately, many of these are segments for whom health care is *not* elastic. They have more serious health problems than average,

HEALTH CARE
✔ HIGHLIGHT

Only 72 percent of Americans were covered by private or government health insurance for the entire 1985-87 period, according to a Census Bureau study.

and they need treatment. The irony of the growing number of uninsured is that most of them work, many at well-paying jobs, and most could easily afford insurance premiums. Unfortunately, an increasing number of employers are dropping health insurance as a benefit, thereby making it prohibitively expensive for the typical wage earner.

An important consideration is the so-called "sandwich" generation, the cohort of baby boomers who are now raising children but are also facing the prospect of having to care for elderly parents. This has not become a widespread phenomenon yet, but as the number of boomers in that situation increases, it will create significant implications for health care consumption.

The diversification of lifestyles has further complicated the health care picture. At one time, physicians and hospitals had a profile of the "good" patient. He followed reasonably appropriate health habits, he trusted the physician, and he paid his bills (or made sure his insurance did). Lifestyle diversity means that the physician never knows what to expect when a patient walks in the door.

The health care consumer of the 1990s is also increasingly likely to be a member of a racial or ethnic minority group. Although minority groups tend to be geographically concentrated, their spreading influence will be felt in many places. Most come from cultural backgrounds that view health and health care from a different perspective. They may not have the same respect for formal institutions that we have developed and, in fact, may distrust any organization that appears to be related to the government. They do not necessarily see the modern American doctor as the appropriate source of care nor contemporary medical and surgical procedures as the appropriate form of treatment. They may have lifestyles and behavior patterns that predispose them to different types of health problems. They are not as likely to participate in traditional insurance programs as yesterday's consumer and, in general, have different needs, perceptions, and behavior regarding the health care system.

Above and beyond demographic considerations, the health care consumer of the 1990s is also different in terms of value orientations. While the quality of care provided will still be important, consumers will be looking for health services provided in a manner that is compatible with their lifestyles. This means they want care that is convenient, expeditiously provided, cost effective, and personable. Bedside manner and the quality of the service provided will be increasingly important. There will be emphasis not on receiving the most expensive or the highest level of care, but on obtaining the "best" level of care. To many consumers, this means the least intrusive form of care. Many consumers are now well informed, and they are unwilling to turn themselves over to the health care system lock, stock, and barrel. They will demand democratic rather than authoritative health care, and they will insist on actively participating in their health care decisions.

CHAPTER THREE

Health Care Consumption

Health Care: A Growth Industry

The second half of the 20th century has been a period of increasing health care consumption in the U.S. Before World War II, health services were used only as a last resort. People had limited confidence in the abilities of hospitals and physicians and did not consider the availability of health care a major issue. The mechanisms for paying for health care services were limited. This is not to say that the absolute volume of health services use did not increase prior to WWII; it did. The population was growing, and medical advances improved the effectiveness of the health care system.

After World War II, the demand for health services escalated. It was not that the population was sicker—we were healthier than we had ever been—but the newfound affluence and widespread availability of health insurance boosted people's ability to buy health services. Most important, health and health care had become major values in American society. Our fascination with technology and science and the value we place on human life further boosted the interest in health care. Some would argue, in fact, that we had become obsessed with health care and with preserving our health, youth, and beauty. The fact that virtually everyone in U.S. society is under some sort of medical management provides strong support for this contention.

This interest in health care led to increasing use of all types of health services. Traditional physicians and hospitals saw use of their services climb, and new practitioners and services emerged to meet the mushrooming demand. We set standards for the frequency of medical checkups, often without scientific basis. Our admonition to "see your dentist twice a year" is in stark contrast to comparable societies where members seldom brush their teeth. Americans purchase medical equipment and pharmaceuticals at a rate not imagined elsewhere. As a society, we have become so obsessed with health care that we have come to see it as a panacea for physical ailments as well as for mental, spiritual, and even social problems.

The Nature of Health Care Consumption

There are certain aspects of health care consumption that set it apart from consumption patterns in other industries. For one thing, it is noteworthy that there is a signficant discrepancy between health care *needs* and health care *wants*. Based on standard clinical criteria, it is fairly easy to estimate the types and level of health problems characterizing a population, especially if one knows something about its demographic makeup. A population of a certain size and demographic composition can be expected to yield a certain number of hospital admissions, physician office visits, diagnoses, and procedures.

There is not a clear match, however, between the health services a population needs and what it actually uses. This was one of the hard lessons of the 1960s, when social service agencies found that the population being served did not necessarily agree that they needed the services offered. It is ironic that the health care industry, above all others, is the one where those who need the services are not necessarily the ones receiving them and those who do not necessarily need the services are consuming more than their share. This situation has given rise to the maxim that the sicker the population, the fewer the health services they are likely to use; the healthier the population, the more.

Another surprising characteristic of health care consumption is the fact that the demand for health services is extremely elastic. Marketers have often considered medical care the one service for which demand is truly inelastic; i.e., if one is sick, one has to consume services. Not only does this reflect a middle-class bias, it assumes that health care refers only to heroic measures performed in life-threatening situations.

As it turns out, that aspect of health care is a relatively rare occurrence. For every episode requiring life-saving efforts, there are thousands of other health care consumption episodes, many involving individuals who are not even sick.

There is ample evidence to support the elasticity of health care demand. Until recent cost-containment measures were instituted, it was apparent that the level of health services use was a function of the facilities and health professionals available. It was always amazing that a community building a new hospital or recruiting additional physicians suddenly found the demand for hospital care or physician services escalating. When it comes to physician-generated demand, one only needs to look at the extreme variation in the use of physician services from market to market. Is it conceivable that two similar populations in different locations could have such disparate health care needs? The practice patterns of local physicians clearly contribute to this situation of elasticity.

Another example is found in the cost-containment developments of the 1980s. In case after case, the level of health services use (and presumably the level of demand) is highly sensitive to the financial mechanisms available. Improving or reducing the financial support for the use of health services seems to be a major contributor to this elasticity. When insurers introduce copayments and higher deductibles into their insurance plans, the use of health services declines. When financial support is augmented, the use of services increases. An excellent case in point is what happened when insurers started offering coverage for mental disorders (including alcohol and drug abuse). The demand for these services skyrocketed, reaching the point, in fact, that many employers were forced to reduce or eliminate their coverage for these services. It is unlikely that there was a sudden explosion in the need for these services. The need may have been there, but it did not translate into consumer demand until there was a way to pay for it.

The bottom line is that there is no close correlation between the prevalence of health problems in a population and its use of health services. In fact, the type of financing available is a better predictor of the use of health services than epidemiological findings related to the incidence of disease.

Changes in Health Care Consumption

DEMOGRAPHIC TRENDS will influence the demand for health services throughout the 1990s. The progressive aging of the population will shift the demand for health services proportionately from one age group to another. The aging of the population will also contribute to its feminization, as the "excess" of females continues to grow.

Technological developments and changes in financing will also contribute to changing consumption patterns, as procedures that once required extensive hospitalization can be done on an outpatient basis and probably less expensively. Health care providers are likely to emphasize prevention and education. Changing reimbursement patterns will influence the service mix of physicians. The lists below indicate some of the changes that can be anticipated by the end of the 1990s.

By the year 2000, there will be more demand for . . .

✓ **Pediatric services,** as the children of the baby boom require additional care

✓ **Older-adult services,** as the number of middle-aged people grows, especially growth in demand for gynecological and urological services

✓ **"Maintenance" services,** as baby boomers enter a stage of chronic conditions, with growing demand for services ranging from corrective lenses (and radial kerotomy) to menopause support groups

✓ **Geriatric services,** as millions of people become elderly during the decade, with increasing demand for geriatricians, physiatrists, cardiologists, oncologists, and rheumatologists

✓ **Preventive care,** as consumer awareness, governmental guidelines, and reimbursement practices converge to make

▶

this a major component of the health care system

✓ **Fitness and wellness programs,** as the above factors, plus employer mandates, work together to demand healthier lifestyles

✓ **Rehabilitation services,** as the number of disabled individuals increases, society becomes more sensitive to the needs of the disabled, rehabilitation technology advances, government regulations mandate treatment, and reimbursement patterns encourage restoration of productive capabilities.

By the year 2000, there will be less demand for . . .

✓ **Obstetrical services,** as the baby boomlet slopes off and the number of potential mothers declines significantly

✓ **Acute care relative to chronic care,** as the cohorts demanding this care remain small, the temporary exception being the children produced by the baby boomlet

✓ **Invasive surgical procedures,** as technology offers less "heroic" alternatives, patients demand less invasive treatment, and third-party payers demand the cost-effective alternative

✓ **Inpatient psychiatric (including substance abuse) services,** with third-party payers and employers demanding the least disruptive and most cost-effective means of treatment

✓ **Trauma services related to violence and accidents,** as the number of people in age groups responsible for most of these events shrinks

✓ **Invasive diagnostic tests,** as various scanning techniques become more common and and microtechnology changes the procedures for internal diagnoses.

The Future of Health Care Consumption

The future of health care consumption will be shaped by the changing character of the health care consumer. The demand for traditional hospital services will increase as the baby-boom generation ages. That phenomenon, however, will not affect hospitals until at least the end of the decade. The hospital population will be sicker and probably more female-dominated. Consumers will also be better informed and will make greater demands for service and information than they have in the past. By then, the challenge may be to find ways to keep certain patients *out* of the hospital. Most hospitals already lose money on Medicare patients and, as other third-party payers follow suit, the situation can only get worse.

Focusing on hospital patients may actually be irrelevant. While it is true that the population will continue to grow (albeit slowly) and to age, these developments do not hold the hope for hospitals that many believe. There are many forces operating to restrict hospitalization, and it is not unrealistic to forecast stability or even continued decline nationally in patient admissions.

If it is not hospital care that people will be consuming, what will it be? The number of hospital admissions is expected to be around 30 million in 1995. In that same year, there will be an estimated 750 million physician office visits, 150 million general physical examinations, 40 million mammograms, and 20 million individuals participating in supervised weight reduction programs. Not only will there be many times more nonhospital episodes than hospital episodes, but the *potential* number of hospital admissions is relatively inelastic. That is, it will be nearly impossible to increase the number of hospital admissions. On the other hand, the demand for nonhospital services is highly elastic and perhaps insatiable.

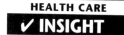

HEALTH CARE

✔ INSIGHT

Because the U.S. population is growing slowly, the overall demand for health care is not increasing dramatically.

Those who consume health care will be less likely to suffer from acute conditions and more likely to suffer from chronic conditions, and chronic conditions generally do not require hospitalization. Compare a 1995 projection of 6 million tonsillectomies (acute condition) with 60 to 100 million treatment episodes for arthritis. The comparisons are endless and underscore the importance of outpatient care and chronic care for the future.

What does this mean for health care consumption for 2000 and the years beyond? Short of a major restructuring of American health care and the reorientation of our nation's values, the health care consumption boom should continue through the 1990s into the next century. There appears to be no limit on the demands consumers are willing to place on the health care system and no limit to the goods and services that the industry can develop to meet these demands. Although we have become more realistic about the benefits of high-tech responses and the ability of formally structured institutions to meet our needs, we still turn to health care for solutions, even if it means taking over our own therapy. Despite efforts at capping the expansion of the health care industry, the forces that operate today will cause it to continue to grow past the turn of the century.

Consumer Decision Making in Health Care

Consumers for many types of health services face a more complex decision-making process than do consumers of most other goods. If it were as simple as one-gets-sick-and-goes-to-the-doctor, it would be different, but it is not. A variety of factors come into play at all stages of the process, from awareness of a need to consumption to repeat use.

It should be noted that health services can be divided into *nonelective,* or urgent, services and *elective* services. Nonelective services are those that are not truly very elastic. They include emergency services and procedures that must be performed to save a patient's life or prevent further serious damage. Elective procedures are those performed for conditions that are not life threatening and, in a sense, are nice to have but are not essential.

The category into which some services fall is debatable, and a lot depends on who is making the decision. Many would consider knee surgery for a professional tennis player as essential and nonelective; for most people, it might be considered elective, assuming that the individual had a reasonable level of mobility. As we have shifted from a medical care orientation to a health care orientation, the variety of elective services has increased, and the proportion of elective health care has grown.

From a marketer's perspective, this is good news. For nonelective procedures, the marketer has limited influence in the decision-making process. But elective procedures offer a wide-open field for the marketer to influence where they are used and who provides them.

Contrary to popular belief, health care consumers go through the same steps in the decision-making process as consumers of other goods. They become aware of a need, they decide that it is important enough to address, they begin an internal and external search for answers to that need, they compare possible sources of services, and they make a decision. Further, they evaluate the quality of services and the outcome, they pass on their evaluation to others, and they decide (if appropriate) whether or not to use those services again. The more elective the procedure is, the more the process resembles that for other consumer goods and services.

This outline oversimplifies the process for health care decision making in the sense that the end user, the patient, may not be the one making all of the decisions. Physicians make some of the decisions, and of course, their criteria for decision making are likely to be different from those of the patient.

It is important to distinguish between correlation and causation when examining health behavior. It is a lot easier to demonstrate correlation than causation. The case for the latter must be much stronger. Ultimately, the marketer may be able to get by with correlating health behavior with various characteristics. In most cases, the marketer does not particularly care why the health care consumer behaves the way he does, just so that he behaves in a predictable manner. The sections that follow outline some of the factors that have been associated with health behavior.

Biological Factors.   At first blush, one would think that biological factors play a highly significant role in health behavior. After all, health problems are essentially biological problems, so there should be a reasonable correlation between morbidity and health care decision making. Males and females may have different health problems as a result of biological differences, as do blacks and whites, and the young and the old. Yet, as noted above, this correlation is not nearly as clear as one would think. Even at the early stages of the process (e.g., perceiving a need, evaluating its seriousness), one person's pathology may be another's normal state. Many people, for example, assume that certain conditions such as chronic fatigue and back pain are a normal part of life and would not consider seeking care for them. Some biological factors do come into play, but these are often overridden by other factors.

Psychological Factors. Psychological factors include personality types and traits, attitudes, and psychoanalytic traits linked to the id, ego, and superego. The relationship between these factors and health behavior can become exceedingly complex, as seen in the case of the hypochondriac or in cases where fear pushes one person to seek treatment but keeps another away from the physician. In the contemporary U.S. health care environment, fear, pride, and vanity play a large role in the demand for many elective procedures (e.g., cosmetic surgery, stomach resection). Psychological factors, while often overshadowed by some of the other factors discussed, play a role at each step in the consumer decision-making process. These are the factors that often play a role in patient satisfaction levels (and often provide disgruntled patients with the basis for a malpractice suit).

Demographic Factors. Although it is difficult to establish a causative link between many demographic variables and health behavior, it is here perhaps that the correlations are best established. Many demographic traits prove to be strong predictors of both the level of health services used and the types of services desired. As noted earlier, these include such traits as age, sex, and even race and ethnicity. Like psychological traits, demographic characteristics play a role at each step of the consumer decision-making process. They are particularly well correlated with the individual's knowledge, attitudes, and preferences about health care.

Social Structural Factors. Health care decision making is influenced by social structural factors in a number of ways, most directly through the effects of marital status, family structure, and household characteristics. Health care decisions are seldom made by individuals;

Goods and Services Consumed During a Hospital Stay

THE FOLLOWING GOODS and services are typically consumed (i.e., purchased) during a hospital stay involving any significant surgical procedure. Some services (i.e., those in the room/board category) are usually included in the daily room charge levied by the hospital. Virtually all other goods and services are charged to the patient separately. Some of the charges are included on the hospital bill (referred to as technical services), and some are charged to the patient separately by physicians and other health professionals (referred to as professional services).

The different departments and personnel involved in the treatment of a hospitalized patient result in a highly complicated system of charges. It is a challenge to ensure that all goods and services are promptly charged to the patient's account. From the patient's perspective, the bills arriving from a variety of sources related to one hospital episode create considerable confusion (especially when different payers are responsible for different charges). The list of goods and services below is not exhaustive, but includes the core of services provided to a surgery patient.

Room/Board

Nursing services
Food services

Physician Services

Attending physician
Surgeon(s)
Consulting specialist
Anesthesiologist
Radiologist
Pathologist

Surgical Services

Operating-room time
Surgical supplies
Attendants/orderlies

Diagnostic Services

Routine lab tests
Pathology lab tests
Routine radiology tests
Special radiology tests (e.g., MRI)
Special diagnostics (e.g., endoscopy)
Monitoring devices (e.g., telemetry)
Emergency physician

▶

Products Purchased	Therapeutic Services
Pharmaceuticals	Respiratory therapy
Medical supplies	Physical therapy
Medical equipment	Speech therapy
Prosthetic devices	Enterostomy therapy
Intravenous solutions	Occupational therapy
Blood & blood components	

Counseling Services	Followup Services/Goods
Social work	Rehabilitation services
Psychological services	Skilled nursing services
	Custodial care
Miscellaneous Services	Home health services
Telephone	Medical equipment
Television	
Cot	

they are often group decisions. Individuals are influenced by their signficant others (hence the importance of marital status) and by the social groups with which they relate. Health consumer decisions are guided by groups of various types. These may be groups to which the individual belongs (such as a religious congregation) or reference groups from which the individual takes his cues (such as a social stratum to which he aspires). Numerous studies have found that choices of treatment reflect the influence of social groups more than obvious factors such as the type of health problem.

Factors Influencing Consumption in the 90s

The 1990s will see certain changes in health care consumption, some of which will bear little relationship to changes in need. Technological developments will continue to influence the consumption of health services. Not only have the advances of the past few years made many procedures considered "impossible" in the past commonplace, but they have changed the nature of the health care setting. Within a decade, surgery was transformed from a strictly inpatient procedure to one more frequently performed in an outpatient setting.

Changing practice patterns on the part of physicians and hospitals will also influence the consumption of health care. Hospitals have already been forced to limit the procedures performed on patients, and changing reimbursement patterns and regulatory pressures are forcing physicians to change their practice patterns as well. These developments will limit the patient's ability to consume certain services in the future.

The big unknown is related to the changes that will occur in the financing of health care during the 1990s. Obviously, there will be continued attempts to reduce expenditures, and patients will be restricted in their ability to receive certain services. However, to the extent that a growing share of services are elective, these regulations will have limited effect. If some form of national health insurance is introduced during this decade, the implications will probably be significant, but it is hard to predict in what ways. A national financing system would surely work to encourage restrictions in the use of care. At the same time, to the extent that it would facilitate the use of services by those who are now excluded from the system, national health insurance could introduce a large number of new consumers into the marketplace.

HEALTH CARE

✔ HIGHLIGHT

By the late 1980s, Medicare was serving more than 22 million people a year, at a cost of more than $70 billion.

The question that should ultimately be asked is: Who will control patients in the 1990s? In actuality, the *real* customers for many health care services in the 1990s will not be individuals at all; they will be organizations. The space on the front sheet reserved for source of referral will less frequently read "Mr." or "Dr." and more frequently read "Inc." While marketers must become increasingly effective in targeting health care's traditional customers (i.e., patients and physicians), they must also develop the means to cultivate third-party payers, employee groups, and other organizations that will control the flow of patients. These issues are discussed in chapter six.

CHAPTER FOUR

Segmenting the Health Care Market

From Mass Marketing to Target Marketing

The most significant development in marketing during the 1980s was the shift from mass marketing to an emphasis on target marketing. By that time, every consumer industry realized that the brand loyalty so highly developed since World War II was giving way to a marketplace demanding custom goods and services. The cultural homogenization that was expected to occur had not happened and, in fact, the population was becoming more heterogeneous in its consumption patterns. Regional differences remained strong, while new ethnic groups were added to the population, and lifestyle differences were more common.

It was no longer sufficient to develop one product (and subsequently one message) for a marketplace that had multiple markets with multiple needs and multiple "hot buttons." Brand image was no longer sufficient for maintaining market share. In fact, major national brands found their market shares eroded by smaller, quicker competitors who were able to tailor their products and messages to capture important niches.

The proliferation of consumer segments means that more research and thought has to go into both product development and promotion. The population has to be subdivided into segments of customers with similar characteristics who are likely to exhibit similar purchase behavior. The needs of each consumer group have to be determined, and successful providers have to respond to these needs. Market segmentation is based on three assumptions: (1) everyone is not a prospect for every product or service, (2) a firm's product/service mix must be controlled for maximum efficiency, and (3) since both product/service mix and the pool of potential customers is limited, efficient operation requires marketing the product in keeping with customer wants and needs. Segmentation, as discussed below, can be based on an almost unlimited number of attributes. The process typically starts with demographic segmentation and works through a number of other dimensions. The complexity of the segmentation and the dimensions that are relevant depend on the industry, of course. In the typical consumer industry, the trend has been to slice and dice the population into ever- smaller segments. This often means that the marketer is focusing on ever-smaller geographic areas. As segmentation increases, one may move from a national market to a regional market to a local market. For many industries, local markets are further subdivided into counties, zip codes, census tracts, and even block groups. With today's direct-marketing technology, it is possible to locate customers at the block-group level. In fact, data are now available down to the household level in some industries, although in most cases, this has limited usefulness for marketing purposes.

Introducing Market Segmentation in Health Care

The development of market segmentation in health care lagged well behind its introduction in other industries. When marketing was introduced into health care during the 1980s, hospitals and other providers essentially took the traditional mass marketing approach that had characterized other industries a decade or two earlier. Hospitals in particular were used to being all things to all people, and they were not easily convinced of the merits of market segmentation and target marketing.

For major producers of health-related goods (e.g., pharmaceuticals and medical supplies), the market was essentially a national one, and for most of these, it remains so today. For hospitals, physicians, and other providers of patient care, it was essentially a local market. The population was seen as a homogeneous group that differed little in its health care needs and consumption patterns. Most providers of health seldom gave any thought to the nature of their markets.

By the late 1980s, health care providers and hospitals in particular were seeing the same sort of erosion in market shares that had happened to market leaders in some other industries. All providers, in fact, were facing increasing competition, and it was not all coming from similar types of providers. True, hospitals were facing stronger competition from other hospitals. But more important, they were being threatened by other types of health care organizations. Minor emergency centers were springing up (to compete with emergency rooms), freestanding diagnostic centers were established (to compete with in-hospital facilities), and outpatient surgery centers were strategically sited (to compete with in-hospital surgical facilities). Even physicians began performing some of the functions historically reserved for hospitals. Physicians themselves began facing stronger competition, from their colleagues, from physicians in other specialties who began encroaching on their turf, and from hospitals who had in the past been their strongest supporters.

Although seldom having the resources of established health care providers, these new competitors were focused and set about capturing niches that cut into the markets of the established providers. The heavy emphasis these providers placed on market research (and the influence that marketing exerted over decision making) allowed them to be more sensitive to changes in consumer purchase patterns and to react to them.

Eventually, it became obvious that the health care market was highly segmented. Different segments were demanding different services tailored to their needs. The demand for services turned out to be more elastic for some segments of the market than for others. It was difficult for conservative hospital administrators to accept that the same factors causing consumers to chose a particular automobile or shampoo were influencing their choices in health care. But that is exactly what was happening.

General Dimensions of Market Segmentation

U.S. society is heterogeneous, and markets can be segmented along any number of dimensions. The basic dimension for market segmentation is demographics, and to a great extent, many other dimensions can be linked back to demographic characteristics. While we all take for granted what demographics is, it is difficult to overstate the complexity of this dimension. Demographic segmentation can be based on age, sex, race, socioeconomic status (e.g., income, industry, education), social structural factors (e.g., marital status, household structure, religion), type of community (e.g., urban, suburban, rural), and any number of other variables. Segmentation becomes even more complex when one considers combinations of these variables. It is one thing to view the consumer behavior of whites and blacks differently, but it becomes more of a challenge when one realizes that segments of lower-income rural whites and upper-income urban blacks exist. This calls for a high level of sophistication in market research and promotional activities.

Life stage is another appropriate basis for consumer segmentation. Depending on one's stage in the life cycle, certain consumer goods and services will be required. Assuming a pattern that involves a progression from dependent youth to college student to young single adult to young married couple to young married couple with children to mature adults with older children to older empty-nesters to senior citizens, it seems reasonable to predict the level and nature of consumer purchases on these grounds.

This manner of segmenting the population has worked fairly well from a marketer's perspective. A certain constellation of goods and services can be linked to each stage. For example, young single adults tend to spend money on cars and alcohol, young marrieds on household goods, young parents on child-related services, and so on. Furthermore, simply knowing someone's age was often a clue to their current life stage.

But traditional patterns no longer hold, and new, more complex patterns are developing. One can no longer assume that the pattern of bachelorhood, marriage, and family formation will be the standard progression. As noted earlier, Americans are more often remaining single, they are marrying later when they do marry, they are having no or fewer children, and the pattern of multiple serial marriages, with all that involves, seems to be well established. As a result, there are few givens in lifecycle progression in today's society.

During the 1980s, two other concepts became popular among marketers. Derived from earlier lifestyle segmentation approaches, the application of psychographic analysis to consumer behavior caught fire.

Lifestyle segmentation appears in two major forms in current marketing research: psychographic schemes and geodemographic cluster systems. Psychographics categorizes consumers based on their values and attitudes. Indeed, the most famous psychographic system incorporates these elements into its name—VALS (Values And Lifestyles System) from SRI International of Palo Alto, California. The second incarnation of VALS—VALS 2—classifies consumers into eight distinct mindsets, including Fulfilleds and Achievers. The system is based on a survey that asks questions like: "Could you stand to skin a dead animal?" Customized VALS surveys then link the attitudinal variables to attitudes and behaviors regarding specific products and services.

Geodemographic cluster systems categorize households rather than people into dozens of lifestyle groups based on demographic and socioeconomic characteristics rather than attitudes. PRIZM, a pioneer geodemographic system from Claritas Corporation of Alexandria, Virginia, has cluster groups with evocative names like "Blue Blood Estates," "Furs and Station Wagons," and "Shotguns and Pickups." Once the households in a specific geographic area (and these can be very small) have been classified, their consumer behavior can be inferred by their similarities to or differences from national norms, based on information from large nationally representative media use and purchase behavior surveys.

Segmentation Dimensions Specific to Health Care

Most standard segmentation dimensions used in other industries apply to health care. The demographic dimensions are all relevant and in fact, probably have more implications for health care than for other consumer industries. As noted previously, one's age, sex and race all can be factors in the types of health problems one faces. This is true for some less obvious demographic variables as well, such as income, education, and industry, and even the type of community one lives in.

Basic biological facts and secondary effects of demographics all contribute to a highly complex segmentation scheme of health care needs.

The situation is more complex when one considers that the demand for health services operates to a certain extent independently of the need for health services. For example, it appears that females in U.S. society consume health services at a rate higher than their level of need seems to dictate. Males, on the other hand, consume services at a rate lower than their level of need suggests. Similarly, blacks typically have higher-than-average health care needs, but they use services at lower-than-average levels. These types of contradictions can be cited repeatedly.

There is a relationship between life stage and health services needs. A different set of needs characterizes young single adults, married adults with young children, married adults with older children, and middle-aged empty nesters. These differences reflect both their structural circumstances (i.e., if you do not have children, you do not use many pediatric services) and the lifestyles and related attitudes and preferences that go along with them. This can be seen in cases where young married couples are very innovative in their choice of health service settings and providers, until they have children. Then, they often revert to a preference for conservative forms of health care.

Despite the relationship between life stage and use of health services, this approach to health care has limitations. For one thing, market research in health care has not developed to the point that there is adequate information on this relationship. The most significant deficiency, however, is the fact that the life-cycle approach is based on the family as the consumption unit, while health services use is a personal thing; one may buy a family car but not a family appendectomy. In any case, health care organizations have not developed mechanisms for householding as other industries have, thereby limiting the applicability of this approach.

Even after hospital marketers accepted the usefulness of market segmentation, the application of psychographic analysis developed slowly. Even those who would have attempted to apply psychographics to health care realized that, as originally formulated, this approach had limited suitability for the industry. Health care consumers were different from the consumers of other goods, and without empirical verification of the relationship between psychographic categories and health care behavior and preferences, it would have been premature to apply existing psychographic frameworks. In addition, health care markets were mostly local markets, and earlier research indicated that health behaviors, preferences, and provider practice patterns varied widely from market to market, something that broad-based national psychographic schemes did not take into account.

By the late 1980s, however, two commercial data vendors had developed lifestyle segmentation systems firmly grounded in health care market research. Using data from a variety of sources—government-sponsored sample surveys, data from registries on facilities utilization, and their own proprietary research—these vendors were able to identify a constellation of health-related behaviors, attitudes, and preferences that could be linked to existing psychographic schemes or to new ones developed specifically for health care.

Health care is also characterized by some dimensions of segmentation that are not significant in other consumer industries, including the consumer's religious affiliation and preference for type of hospital. Hospitals, and increasingly their affiliated providers, are often funded and/ or operated by various religious denominations. Although there does not appear to be a universal preference for health care systems sponsored by the consumer's denomination, in some markets,

HEALTH CARE

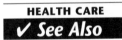 **✔ See Also**

See the appendix on page 173 for sources of psychographic data.

Catholics and Jews would not consider entering any hospital other than Catholic and Jewish hospitals, respectively. In fact, marketers in these areas may be faced with the challenge of convincing non-Catholics and non-Jews that these hospitals are for them, too.

A related issue has to do with the variety of sponsors of health systems. Beyond the religious issue described above, hospitals and other sources of care may be private not-for-profit entities, private for-profit entities, or they may be sponsored by various levels of government. They may be independent and community-based, or they may be operated as part of a national chain. They may be research-oriented, teaching-oriented, profit-oriented, community-service-oriented, or have some other emphasis. In fact, even if they do not officially emphasize any type of health care, consumers may view them as being in a particular category. For example, it is not unusual for a "public" hospital to be considered a place strictly for the indigent and undesirable or a medical-school-affiliated hospital as a place where you may be used as a research subject. Consumers have a variety of perceptions (and misconceptions) related to the quality and acceptability of these facilities. Different segments of the market have different perceptions, and these must be considered when marketing hospitals and related facilities.

Source of Financing.   Marketers typically think of consumers by their income level and segment the market on that basis. Different categories of consumers have varying levels of ability to pay and are thus more or less price sensitive in their consumer decisions. For most consumer products, knowing the level of income and something about the consumer's credit status is adequate for determining ability to pay. This information is available at local levels of geography and provides the basis for much marketing in other industries.

This source-of-financing approach takes an interesting twist in health care. For many health services consumed, consumers themselves are not directly responsible for the costs. Those with extensive insurance coverage may be virtually insulated from the cost aspect of their consumer behavior. Not only are they not responsible for paying the bill, they may not even know what they were charged. In other cases, the end user may be responsible for only part of the bill. This increases the interest and participation of the end user but still keeps him somewhat insulated from the effects of the costs.

Other consumers may have insurance that places limits on reimbursement for various health services. To the extent that the provider can not charge the patient for the shortfall, the consumer once again becomes cost-insensitive. Some people have little or no insurance, and these are the only people who are not insulated from the price aspect of care. They are expected to pay their health care expenses out of pocket. This is a growing group in U.S. society, one that will continue to be problematic for the system. Few uninsured individuals can pay for the entire cost of their health care, resulting in a large segment of medically indigent citizens. On the other hand, the medically indigent often receive essentially free public care, and even *they* become insulated from price.

For these reasons, the type of insurance coverage available is typically a better indicator of the patient's ability to pay than the standard measures of economic status used in other industries. The situation is complicated by the fact that this measure of ability to pay varies depending on the type of service required. Historically, hospital care and other major medical expenses have been covered under insurance programs. Physician care, particularly routine office visits, has been more likely to be paid out of pocket by the consumer. Looked at another way, urgent or nonelective procedures are usually covered under insurance programs, while elective procedures (e.g., cosmetic surgery) are seldom covered. As various third-party payers have taken a more active role in monitoring patient spending, the complexity of the reimbursement situation has increased. Different insurers provide different levels of reimbursement.

Ultimately, the health care marketer needs to segment the market by its ability to pay. This segmentation must then be adjusted in view of the types of services being marketed. When marketing a trendy elective procedure (e.g., tummy tucks), insurance coverage is less of an issue than the patient's level of discretionary income. On the other hand, if one is promoting an open-heart-surgery program, it would be a mistake to market to any segment that was not well insured.

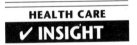

HEALTH CARE

✔ INSIGHT

The significance of health insurance coverage depends on how necessary or elective the health service is.

Other Dimensions. Many health care organizations have attempted to segment consumers on the basis of health problems, categorizing them in terms of specialties or, more recently, product lines. This is a reasonable approach in that a relatively healthy female obstetrics patient has different needs than a very sick elderly oncology patient. Hospitals have been more active in developing product lines than have other providers (although the for-profit purveyors of goods—the pharmaceutical and medical supply firms—have long used a product-line approach). However, the variety of services (and goods) that can be purchased is endless. Many diagnoses do not fit neatly under one spe-

Demographics, Market Segmentation, and Health Care

THREE DECADES of health-services research and epidemiological studies have established a strong association between demographic characteristics and various aspects of health and health care. While it may not be appropriate to contend that certain demographic characteristics *cause* health conditions or influence health behavior, strong links have been demonstrated for many variables.

A number of demographic variables serve as useful predictors of health status. They indicate both the level and type of health problems likely to characterize a particular population. For example, one can profile teenagers, young adults, and senior citizens by how often they report health problems and the types of problems they report. The age distribution of a population thus becomes a strong predictor of health problems.

Sex and race also serve as predictors for level and type of health problems. Women clearly suffer from different types of problems than men, and most studies indicate a higher level of morbidity for women in general (although men experience a higher mortality rate). One can also identify differences in health status between whites and nonwhites, with nonwhites tending to have a greater number and variety of health problems than whites. Blacks in particular suffer from higher prevalence rates for most conditions (both acute and chronic) and suffer more serious cases of those conditions.

Health status in general tends to rise with income, education, and occupational status. Similarly, specific health problems are associated with various income, educational, and occupational categories. Marital status and household

▶

structure are also surprisingly good predictors of health status and type of condition. For example, married people benefit from much better health than those of any other marital status.

The demographic categories noted above serve as good predictors of health-services use just as they do for health status itself. Differences in the use of health services reflect, to a certain extent, the differences in health status noted above. But some demographic traits influence health-services utilization quite apart from actual level of morbidity. People in some demographic categories have a greater propensity to use health services regardless of their health status.

The frequency of use and type of health services used are highly age specific. Physician services tend to be geared to different age groups. Women use different types of services than men, and they use them more often. On the other hand, nonwhites tend to use most services less than whites, despite their higher demonstrated need. They also use different types of services.

Use of health services tends to rise with income, education, and occupational status, despite the fact that those of higher socioeconomic status tend to have better health. And although married individuals tend to be healthier, they also use health services at a higher rate than others.

Demographic characteristics provide useful guidelines for both the incidence of health problems within the population and the level of health-services utilization. Many of these correlations are predictable, but in many other cases, unexpected associations exist between demographic variables and health status and health behavior. Health care marketing can only be effective if these relationships are well understood.

cialty category, and most conditions require services that cut across product lines and specialties. Despite some potential benefits, product-line management has had limited success because the approach essentially structures operations from the perspective of the provider and not from that of the customer.

Some health care organizations are beginning to look at customers by such factors as usage rates and brand loyalty. Different segments display different levels of health care usage. For example, heavy users of minor emergency centers may include affluent working parents and their children, laborers whose employers have arrangements with the center, and newly arrived transferees who have not established a physician relationship. The only thing these groups may have in common is their propensity to use minor emergency centers. Similarly, patients with loyalty to a certain hospital may cut across a number of demographic or other segmentation dimensions. Nevertheless, they should be handled differently than those loyal to other facilities, regardless of the segments in which they fall for other dimensions.

It should be noted that this discussion of market segmentation has related only to the end user, the patient. Chapter six discusses the other kinds of customers health care organizations have. These other customers are also segmented in many ways and have to be approached in a manner similar to patients. They include physicians, employers, business coalitions, and other intermediaries that come between the patient and the provider.

Physicians provide an excellent case for a segmentation approach. They can be divided by specialty, type of practice, activity level, or life stage. Family practitioners have to be approached differently than surgeons, independent practitioners differently than group members, and heavy admitters differently than those loyal to another hospital. Similarly, as hospitals and other providers address the industrial market, they must be able to segment employers on the basis of likely health needs, type of insurance, location, and many other factors. In short, segmentation does not end with the patient. Any group that can be con-

HEALTH CARE

✔ See Also

For more information on marketing to doctors see suggested readings on page 171.

sidered a customer of the health care provider can and should be thought of in terms of segmentation.

Bases for Competition in Health Care

Consumers in most industries can be categorized by the factors ("hot buttons") to which they respond. Marketing literature is full of reports about how different segments of the market respond to different incentives. Some segments are highly price sensitive; their level of consumption is highly elastic in the face of price changes. Other segments are insensitive to price and focus instead on quality. Still others focus on a combination of price and quality, looking for the **value** they perceive themselves to be receiving. The hot buttons for other segments may be convenience, service, location, or some other factor unrelated to either price or quality. In an age of consumer awareness, even factors like environmental responsibility become hot buttons for some consumers.

Not too long ago, when it was assumed that the typical consumer of health services was a well-insured hospital patient, the notion of discussing hot buttons in health care would have been laughable. Conventional wisdom held that health care consumers were sick people who needed expert care. The consumer's main concern was that quality services were provided. After all, his life was at stake.

Quality of care continues to be an important issue with health care consumers, but it has been tempered by other factors. For one thing, market research has found that consumers do not discriminate among comparable institutions by quality of care. For example, if there are three major hospitals in a market, consumers are likely to perceive that their medical staffs, nursing staffs, and levels of technology are essentially equal, or at least meet some minimal standard of quality.

Consumers are not in a particularly good position to evaluate these aspects of the facilities they are using. But they can evaluate lots of other factors. Health care consumers are increasingly sensitive to the **service** they receive. This may refer to how the hospital nurses treated the family, how easy admission registration was, how understandable the bill was, and how timely the food service was. Hospitals that made their reputations with high-tech equipment are finding that today's customers are less interested in high tech than they are in high touch. They are not so much interested in whether or not the hospital has the latest multi-million device, but whether the patient's family was made comfortable during the stay. Similarly, physicians are finding that their patients are more likely to sue them over a failure to communicate with them in a personal manner than they are over a clinical mistake. In fact, upstart competitors have often carved out a niche by offering the personal service that many hospitals and physicians did not. What patient would return to a hospital emergency room once the nurse at the minor emergency center called the next day to personally check on his condition? Thus, good service becomes a competitive advantage.

Consumers also increasingly evaluate health care organizations in terms of **amenities**. When market research on health care consumers was first conducted in the 1980s, hospital administrators were shocked to find that consumers were choosing the competitor's hospital because the parking was more convenient or because the rooms were better appointed. Even more shocking was the fact that respondents on patient surveys indicated that Hospital A had the best doctors for their particular problem, but that they would actually use Hospital B when it came time to be admitted. They explained this by saying that it would be easier for their families to visit them at Hospital B or because Hospital B had a senior program that offered their families a cafeteria discount. The less life-threatening the situation, the more important amenities are.

HEALTH CARE

✔ INSIGHT

Patients cannot evaluate the quality of care they receive as well as they can rate the amenities provided.

Health care consumers are also looking for something that could be categorized as **convenience**. Other industries had spoiled consumers by taking their services to the people. Hospitals responded to this sort of need in the 1970s and 1980s by following consumers into the suburbs. Physicians, dentists, and other office-based practitioners also went to the desirable patients. These moves were steps in the right direction, but what today's health care consumer wants is convenience not only in location, but hassle-free processing, quick service, easy financial arrangements, and efficient case managment. These needs have been bolstered by demographic changes such as two working parents.

Locational issues relate not only to physical distances but to social distances as well. Today's consumers want a setting for health services delivery that they are comfortable with and can relate to. In order to attract a certain type of clientele, not only does the facility have to be appropriately located, but its design and operation have to reflect the orientation of the consumers it hopes to serve.

One other issue that should be noted is the modern health care consumer's need to maintain some level of **control** of the process. The naïve dependent patient has been replaced by a better-informed, more assertive customer. As the control-oriented baby-boom cohort makes its presence felt in health care, this aspect of service can only become more important. Consumers want information that will allow for better decision making. Knowledge is power, and today's health care consumer is determined to become empowered.

These changed expectations do not stop with the patients themselves. It should be remembered that those paying the bill, particularly employers, also have expectations. They may not be quite as concerned about the oriental rugs in the waiting room as their employees are, but after quality of care, they want good service for themselves and their employees. They want their employees to stay well, and they want them to be processed in an efficient manner. They want providers to be responsive to their needs as payers and to their employees' needs as end users.

One note of caution: be careful not to overgeneralize. Health care consumers have changed a lot, but they are not a homogeneous market. True, the contemporary well-informed consumer may emphasize convenience, efficiency, and value, but not all consumers fall into this category. Most older Americans—a group with significant health care needs—are responsive to other hot buttons. They are more likely to emphasize quality of care, state-of-the-art equipment, and traditional forms of service. Various ethnic groups may react differently to different aspects of care, and these aspects have to be considered in both product development and marketing.

Implications for Health Care Marketing

The segmented nature of the health care market has a number of important implications for health care marketing. The situation further underscores the need to know the consumer; it calls for a detailed appreciation of the consumer's characteristics and expectations. It further emphasizes the need to move from an emphasis on physical facilities to an emphasis on services. In today's environment, it is no longer appropriate simply to sell bricks and mortar; health care consumers and those paying their bills want results.

To carry this idea further, these trends call for an emphasis on relationships between providers and their customers. Buildings and equipment will not solve health problems any more than school buildings and chalk will solve educational problems. It is the quality of the process that must be emphasized, not the size of the hospital.

These developments mean that providers will have to get better at tailoring their services to the consumer. Only now are hospitals and other health care providers going to the consumer to find out what he needs, rather than trying to force square services into the round hole of consumer desires. It also means that the mechanisms for reaching the consumer have to be modified. Traditional media advertising loses much of its effectiveness in the face of the market segmentation described above. Only by using direct marketing can one tap the potential of this highly differentiated market. Only with database marketing can a provider keep up with and service his customers.

Perhaps the most important reason to segment the health care market is the growing need to identify and manage customers who constitute a number of submarkets. One trend emerging in health care is the development of "customer line management," "customer segment management," or some similar concept built on the recognized segmentation of the health care market. Customer segment management takes an approach quite contrary to the product-line management that has become popular with some hospitals. It identifies segments among the organization's customers and among the general public that can be "managed" in such a way to capture much of their health care business.

A customer segment could be any subgroup within the population that has a set of characteristics and perhaps unique needs. Whatever the needs of the segment are, they are likely to cut across a variety of product lines or specialties, across a variety of settings for care, and involve a number of different circumstances. From this perspective, an important customer segment might be women of childbearing age. In this case, an obvious need is for obstetrical and gynecological services. After all, women in this category use services at a higher rate than just about any other nonelderly segment. But their needs do not end at the OB/GYN department. They are likely to need associated services such as nutritional information, fitness programs, and perhaps psychological services. Further, after childbirth, they will require pediatric services and perhaps other nonmedical services for small children.

Although many of these services are obtained in the form of OB/GYN services, others are physician-office based, hospital based, and in some other setting. In short, the constellation of needs characterizing this group extends across specialties and care settings. Any number of similar customer segments can be identified, such as older adults, the young old, adolescents, and so forth.

A customer-segment approach differs from a product-line approach in some important ways. The key to the customer-segment approach is that it views health services from the perspective of the consumer. Health care consumers do not, unless they are forced to, view health services in narrow categories. They present a need that requires a continuum of services crossing many traditional structural boundaries. They expect a "package" of services that comprehensively meets their needs. The product-line approach actually works in the opposite manner. It tends to make existing structural differences more rigid by focusing inward on a specific product-line such as cardiology, neurosciences, or obstetrics. The organizational structure becomes more vertical at a time when the customer is looking for horizontal integration. Perhaps the most damning aspect of the product-line approach is that it organizes services in a manner convenient for the provider. The rationale behind product-line development is to enhance internal control and introduce efficiencies into the provision of an isolated set of services. Even when its supporters point to it as a framework for marketing, it still ends up as a benefit for the hospital and not for its customers.

···
From Consumer to Customer

"Many industries are dealing with markets that are not grow-ing and are saturated with competition. You must substitute growth in knowledge about your customers for growth in the number of customers."

—Brad Edmondson, author, *Health Care Consumers*

Why Marketing Health Care Is Different

A marketer exposed to the health care industry for the first time will be struck by the differences between health care marketing and the mar-keting of other goods and services. It is true that certain segments of the health care industry approximate other industries in their marketing techniques. These include such for-profit sectors as pharmaceuticals and medical-equipment suppliers for which the business-to-business marketing aspects are similar to those in other industries.

When it comes to marketing to the end user, the patient, manifold differences are apparent. The marketer quickly realizes that health care marketing requires different approaches and messages. Most impor-tant, health care marketing requires a different mind-set than marketing in any other industry. In fact, health care marketing is still in an embry-onic stage, and many techniques demanded by the differences charac-terizing this industry are still being developed. The sections below summarize some of the reasons why health care marketing is different than marketing in other industries.

Nature of the industry.   The health care industry is highly frag-mented with a variety of care providers that often operate autono-mously and without direct interface with many other parts of the indus-try. The channels for consumer entry into health care are numerous and contribute to the complexity. As an industry, health care has no estab-lished pricing mechanisms, and in fact, its whole financing setup is chaotic. Patients often pay very different prices for the same services.

Nature of the consumer.   The health care consumer is a clear anomaly among the purchasers of goods and services. Because of the nature of health care, the use of health services is an emotional issue; the individual's well-being, quality of life, and even life itself may be at stake. Despite this, health care consumers are probably less informed than consumers in any other industry. They are isolated from decision making to a great extent and from the financial aspects as well. Their motivations for the use of health care vary widely, compared with con-sumer behavior in other industries, and they are driven by everything from fear to vanity. The consumption of many types of health services is a rare event for most consumers. Most people buy cars more often than they go to the hospital, and some buy cars more often than they see a physician.

Nature of the product.   One of the first questions asked by market-ers when they began entering the health care arena was: What are you selling? This started a major debate in health care that has not yet been resolved. For providers of care, defining their "product" is extremely difficult. In the for-profit goods-producing sector, the product is fairly clear-cut. For the hospital or physician, on the other hand, the product could be any number of things. The nature of health care almost pre-cludes a product orientation, yet marketing demands that one be able to identify specific products that one wants to deliver.

Nature of decision making.   The consumer decision-making pro-cess in health care is different than that of any other industry. When the end user, the patient, is the decision maker, his decisions are often driven by factors that have little to do with his health condition. The consumer behavior process may be influenced by social factors, demo-graphic considerations, attitudes or emotions, or a variety of other

A Marketer in Health Care Land

WHEN HEALTH CARE organizations began turning to marketing during the mid-1980s, they typically turned to other industries for marketing professionals. At that time, virtually no one had been trained in health care marketing, so it was necessary to look to such industries as financial services and hospitality for marketing expertise.

It is safe to say that virtually every marketer entering health care from another industry underwent culture shock. Health care organizations, with a few exceptions, had never had a marketing orientation and were not consumer-driven. There was little in the way of existing market intelligence, market research techniques in the industry were poorly developed, and the techniques in other industries had limited application to health care.

Take the example of a marketer who comes to health care from the restaurant industry. On the surface, there are some similarities between health services and food services. Both serve customers with clearly identified needs and provide goods and/or services that are generally tailored to the needs of the customer.

But if the marketer views a hospital as a fast-food restaurant, what does he find? The first thing he realizes is that customers at the hospital typically did not come of their own accord; someone else (e.g., a physician) sent them there. Furthermore, when they got to the hospital, there was no menu of services to choose from; someone else (again, usually a physician) chose the services for them.

To the extent that the patient/customer does know what services are available, she is typically not aware of the prices, similar to an upscale restaurant that has no prices listed on the menu. This doesn't matter either, since someone else will probably be paying the bill. One reason that pricing is a problem is because

▶

the hospital has little idea of what to charge for its services. Its administrators typically do not know what it costs to produce a service, and they usually do not know what their competitor down the street is charging for the same service. Hospitals consider pricing proprietary information and generally do not make it available unless mandated by regulatory agencies to do so.

What may really surprise the marketer is that the cooks (the physicians) at this restaurant (the hospital) do not even work for the organization. They are independent operators who come in, use the restaurant's facilities (free of charge), and charge the customers for their services independent of what the restaurant charges. The restaurant, in this analogy, charges only for the use of the tables and chairs, and the consumption of condiments and napkins, but the cooks charge for the actual food provided. Even more surprising is the fact that the cooks tell the customers (the patients) what to order, how long they should stay at the restaurant, and when they should come back.

The customer is not in a position to debate the choices made by the cook and, in fact, is not really allowed to question the appropriateness or the quality of the services provided. If a customer were so bold as to do that, the cook is likely to respond: "So what cooking school did you attend?" At the conclusion of the transaction, the cook will indicate when the customer should return for more services and maybe even what the customer should do between "visits." Even if the customer does not agree, she is pretty much bound to comply.

In short, the health care marketer is faced with a unique situation in which someone else may determine the customer's needs, the customer is unaware of the services available, the customer typically is not price-sensitive, and the two parties providing services (hospitals and physicians) not only operate relatively independently, but charge the customer separately. Aside from these factors, the health care marketer can proceed as in any other industry.

factors that have little to do with the actual health care needs of the individual. In actuality, though, the end user is often not the prime decision maker. For example, the woman of the house is usually the decision maker when it comes to initiating health care; she determines what the appropriate decision is and where the care should be obtained, even for her spouse and children. The physician also makes important decisions for the consumer, and this authority is now being shared by employers, insurers, and other third-party payers who are trying to exert some control over costs.

Because of these factors, the challenges facing a health care marketer are of a greater magnitude than those facing marketers in industries where the nature of the consumer and the product lend themselves to a more traditional marketing orientation. It should be noted, however, that all is not lost. Health care marketing does, in fact, have some characteristics in common with marketing in other industries.

How Health Care Marketing Is Similar

Health care consumers are still consumers.   Despite their unique characteristics, the consumers of health services share many characteristics with consumers of other goods and services. They go through much the same general process of problem identification, search for solutions, evaluation of options, purchase behavior, and post-purchase evaluation. They develop preferences for certain types, locations, and modes of health services. They are heavily influenced by their past experiences, the input of friends and relatives, and expert advice. They have certain expectations about quality, service, and outcomes, although the slant on each is somewhat different in health care. Like all consumers, they have certain triggers that indicate when consumption should occur, although these triggers are surprisingly different from one segment of the population to another.

Social factors play a major role in the decision-making process.
Given the nature of health problems, one would think that practical considerations related to the nature of the problem and the appropriate services would be the main factors in deciding to seek treatment, in choosing the type of care (e.g., chiropractor versus orthopedic

surgeon), in choosing the particular physician, in selecting a hospital, and in complying with a doctor's orders. In reality, the nature of the problem has less to do with these decisions than do the demographic, psychographic, and socioeconomic attributes of the affected individual. In fact, medical sociologists have found that the decision to seek treatment usually results because the condition is interfering with interpersonal relationships and/or social role performance. People often tolerate extreme pain, discomfort, and personal dysfunction without seeking treatment as long as it does not interfere with their social functioning. Untold numbers of very sick people have put off seeking treatment because they did not want to inconvenience the family, did not trust doctors, could not afford the treatment, would be embarrassed in front of their friends, or any number of other reasons that have nothing to do with the health problem itself.

Health care consumption is predictable. In the past, many observers have indicated that the use of health services is unpredictable. Catastrophic illnesses are rare and unpredictable events, as are major accidents. Many conditions appear without warning (e.g., appendicitis), while others linger unnoticed, only to surface in response to some unpredictable trigger (e.g., AIDS). However, these rare events actually account for only a small portion of health care consumption, and few are truly unpredictable. Even accidents, which one would assume to be the most unpredictable of health-related events, can be predicted within reason. With the information we have available today, health care planners can determine for a given population the expected number and type of accidents and how they will be distributed by the victims' characteristics. The same is possible for virtually every other condition.

Health care consumption is elastic. The level of health care consumption is surprisingly elastic, sensitive to a variety of factors unrelated to health problems themselves. While certain urgent conditions will almost always result in treatment, within a population as complex as that of the U.S., the consumption of a particular health service may vary even if actual need is held constant. For example, the share of people who go for a regular physical exam varies widely based on demographic characteristics. Presumably, the need for a regular checkup is uniform throughout the population, but women get them more often than men, whites more often than blacks, the affluent more often than the poor. Furthermore, these levels of use tend to change under certain conditions even without any obvious change in demographic or socio-economic factors—for example, when insurance is provided for a certain service or when new facilities or services are offered where there were none before. The elasticity is further demonstrated by the fact, as seen below, that consumption of health services may be faddish, with patients and physicians alike taking off on "popular" procedures. As the proportion of elective procedures increases, one can expect more elasticity in the demand for health services.

Health care consumption is faddish.   As surprising as it may seem, both patients and physicians are susceptible to fads in the use of health services. While faddishness on the part of consumers is likely to be restricted to situations in which they have ample control, physicians have been found to be susceptible even when the procedures are related to life-threatening situations. In recent years, for example, doctors have performed cesarean sections on pregnant women more often than the clinical situation demands. The rate of cesarean sections soared during

HEALTH CARE

✔ HIGHLIGHT

Between 1980 and 1988, the cesarean-section rate grew 40 percent, from 5.3 per 1,000 population to 7.4 per 1,000.

the 1970s and 1980s until certain observers began questioning the necessity of this nontrivial procedure. Similarly, at various times, it has been faddish to routinely remove children's tonsils or to insert ear tubes. Physicians, as it turns out, are human and are susceptible to the same factors that influence the rest of us. Consumers also frequently pursue trendy types of care. How could the tremendous jump in the patronage of psychiatrists during the 1960s be explained otherwise? This was not a decade of widespread insanity, but a time when it was popular to have a "shrink."

Health care consumer segments have hot buttons.   Only recently have market researchers in health care come to realize that health care consumers respond to certain issues in much the same way as consumers of other goods. Certainly, sick people are concerned about the efficacy of the treatment they receive, but beyond some minimal level of assurance about the outcome, health care consumers are often sensitive to considerations totally unrelated to the quality of care. This fact becomes more apparent as patients take a more active role in decision making and as the share of elective procedures grows.

Although the particular "hot buttons" differ from market segment to market segment, health care consumers respond to location, convenience, efficiency, personableness, prestige, or certain amenities associated with the facility or practitioner. Patients, in fact, are not well qualified to judge the quality of physician care or nursing care, nor can they really assess the appropriateness of a medical outcome. They can evaluate how pleasantly and efficiently they were processed, whether the hospital room was nicely decorated, how good the food was, and how convenient the parking or the doctor's hours were. These factors are increasingly influencing consumer behavior, and the marketer must be able to link them to various services and market segments.

The "Missing Links" of Health Care Marketing

Marketers entering any industry have certain expectations about the resources "in place" to facilitate marketing. These expectations include a certain knowledge base, established product attributes, a rational pricing structure, and some tried-and-proven marketing techniques. Virtually none of these marketing prerequisites exists in health care, particularly in the components related to patient care. The sections below describe some of these "missing links" in health care and their implications for marketing.

Market Intelligence.   The ability of health care organizations to develop market intelligence in the past has been totally inadequate and is still limited today. Standard market research techniques have limited application in health care, and new techniques are only now being developed. Although the industry was drowning in data, much of the information was useless for market research purposes. The data that existed were internally generated and usually proprietary. Except in the few cases where local health planning agencies compiled data from a variety of providers, there was no public source of market intelligence. A lack of data on physician practices was especially noteworthy.

Health care administrators had almost no understanding of how consumers behaved or why. They could not describe their own patients, much less the general consumer population. Only with the introduction of competition in the mid-1980s did market research activity increase. Hospitals and other providers suddenly needed data on the market and their existing patients. They began to conduct primary research or engage market research firms to do it. A new industry developed devoted to research on the health care consumer.

Well-defined "products."   One assumption in the marketing process is that the product or service to be marketed is well defined and clearly delineated. In contrast, the notion of "product" in health care was unknown until the 1980s. Indeed, one of the first issues that confronted marketers entering health care was the delineation of health care products. The responses to the question of what a provider provides were numerous and disparate. Is the product a particular procedure (e.g., an appendectomy or an x-ray), a good (e.g., a pill or crutches), or a service (e.g., physical therapy or room service)? Is the product something more amorphous, such as an effective outcome (e.g., a cure or restored functioning) or, more amorphous yet, something like "quality of life" or "health?" All of these are products from someone's perspective, and these examples indicate the extensiveness and complexity of product delineation in this industry.

Established marketing techniques.   When marketing met health care, there were no established techniques for marketing to consumers in the industry. Any "marketing" that had occurred in the past had essentially taken the form of public relations and community relations. This void was initially filled by the marketer's standby—advertising. Hospitals in particular turned to newspapers, magazines, radio, television, and billboards in an attempt to attract customers. The application of standard marketing (*read* advertising) techniques to health care resulted in millions of dollars in spending, but with little else to show for it.

Health care consumers are different, and they require different marketing techniques. Marketers had to learn that the market for health care was not a mass market, that image was not as important as service, that patients are not the ones making many of the buying decisions, and that third-party payers greatly complicate the health care consumption process. They had to learn that health care consumers respond to different triggers than do other consumers. The new cadre of health care marketers were slow to learn this because health care administrators did not really understand these issues themselves.

Not only were there no techniques for marketing to the health care consumer, health care was light years behind other industries in marketing to organizations. The concept of marketing to physician groups or groups of purchasers was unprecedented, and no methods had been developed. Yet, as the 1980s unfolded, it became obvious that standard consumer marketing techniques were less and less effective in reaching the parties that really mattered.

Further, no standards existed to measure the effectiveness of marketing activities. The usual measures from other industries were not very useful. Standard indicators such as the number of exposures, top-of-mind awareness, positive perceptions, and so forth were not necessarily indicators of marketing success in health care, especially when they did not translate into bottom-line use of the facility. What was the marketer to think when consumers thought first of the client hospital, preferred it over all others, and considered it to have the best medical staff, but when it came time to be hospitalized, chose some other facility?

A rational pricing structure.   Marketers typically expect to be able to operate within the framework of a rational pricing structure for the goods and services being marketed. While health care organizations do not often compete on price, and consumers often do not know what prices health care providers charge, some rational pricing mechanism is important in positioning a product or service in the marketplace. Marketers found that few health care providers could calculate how much it cost them to provide a service, making it difficult to establish an appropriate price. Further, it was impossible to compare prices of a client institution with competitor institutions because the data from respective institutions were not comparable, assuming they were even available. Many marketers found themselves in the position of heavily marketing a service that was not even profitable.

Rational financing arrangements.   Marketers assume that certain knowledge exists about the financial arrangements of customers in any industry. The situation for health care, however, is quite complex. Customers may pay for different services in different ways, different customers may pay for the same services in different ways, many customers have multiple sources of payment for the services they receive, and some customers cannot pay at all for the services they consume.

For the marketer, this means that there are patients and then there are patients. Marketers may generate a great deal of demand for a particular service, only to find out that users of that service do not have a favorable payer mix. Complicated financial arrangements introduce another dimension into the segmentation process and demand a greater variety of "packages" to meet these disparate consumer needs.

These barriers to developing a true marketing orientation are being partly addressed today. On one hand, health care providers are attempting to define the range of products they offer, and as they develop and/or repackage services, they are applying this product orientation. Health care providers are trying to determine the costs involved in producing various services so they can introduce a more rational pricing approach. They are also involved in reorganizing their internal data management procedures in an effort to generate meaningful data.

On the other hand, health care marketers are busily adapting marketing techniques from other industries. The growing health data industry is filling some of the marketing intelligence gaps and developing techniques to acquire and manage health data.

Finding the Health Care Customer

Once the marketer understands the characteristics and needs of the health care consumer, the next job is to find the customer. Most, if not all, individuals are potential customers. The trick is to turn some portion of the mass of consumers into *your* customers. The process is similar to other consumer industries, but health care marketers may have to modify and add steps to effectively locate the health care customer. The steps follow:

• ***Profile target customers.*** The first step is to develop a profile of the ideal customer for a particular service. Essentially, one must determine the characteristics of the likely customer for this service. As in other industries, the customer is profiled by demographic characteristics, socioeconomic characteristics, and attitudes.

A typical approach is to profile existing users of a particular service. These patients should be profiled by the characteristics noted above, as well as by source of payment, relevant clinical variables, physician relations, and any other important factor. Information about these patients should indicate the prototype patient to be sought out in the general population.

HEALTH CARE

✔ INSIGHT

Health care marketers initially attempted to identify the ideal customer for a particular institution, but found that consumers and physicians do not buy institutions; they buy specific services.

It is important to carefully examine the characteristics of existing patients, because some subgroups are "better" patients than others (for example, by their ability to pay). In fact, it could be possible that the "wrong" types of patients are actually being attracted to this service. For example, childbirth classes may attract a number of indigent women who expect to deliver their babies at the facility, although they have limited ability to pay.

If the service being offered is new, the marketer must develop a profile of likely patients from some other source. It may be possible to determine the characteristics of the users of these services at other facilities, but since the facilities may be competitors, this information may be hard to come by. More likely, the marketer will have to determine the profile from national data based on facilities where the service is offered. If the new service is truly innovative, it may be necessary to speculate about the characteristics of likely users.

Assuming that the characteristics of existing patients are satisfactory, the marketer can use this profile to "clone" additional patients in the general population. The challenge is to locate and cultivate those potential consumers who are not now using the service or who are customers of a competitor.

This process involves anticipating what consumers want. But how does one determine this? A place to start is with national or regional trends that will affect everyone (including your patients). These trends may be demographic, social, economic, or even technological in nature. The most significant demographic trend, and one that has been referred to often before, is the aging of the population. As baby boomers move into their late 40s, their health care needs are changing dramatically. Today, this gigantic population cohort needs obstetrical and pediatric services; soon, it will demand gynecological and urological services. OB/GYNs with large obstetrical practices now need to position themselves to capitalize on the growing gynecological market of tomorrow.

Social trends, often unrelated to developments in medicine, also must be anticipated. As discussed in chapter two, health care consumers are becoming better educated and, led by the control-oriented baby boomers, are demanding a greater role in their own health care. Physicians and hospitals that can "catch the wave" will find an eager clientele; those that do not may face a dwindling patient population. These "new" patients want information from the physician, and they want to be able to have some input. Physicians and hospital administrators will have to adapt to this new orientation. Other responses to social trends may include restructuring office hours, introducing new services or procedures, and creating marketing initiatives to tell the customer that your practice is state-of-the-art. The fitness boom of the 1980s demonstrated how a social trend could have significant implications for health care.

Economic trends with implications for customers relate principally to the impact of insurance and other third-party payers on the demand for health care. The services customers demand are driven in part by what their insurance pays for. Who could have anticipated the demand for psychiatric services and substance-abuse programs that emerged when these conditions were first covered by private insurance? Even a relatively simple development, such as Medicare's decision to cover the cost of mammograms for women, dramatically changed the demand structure for that diagnostic procedure. Economic trends also may relate to the workplace and the increasing role that the employer is playing in the health care system. Changing economic conditions in the industrial sector have led to a demand for employee-assistance programs, health and safety programs, on-site health facilities, and a number of other programs related to industrial health.

Technological breakthroughs often result in significant changes in health care. While the role of technology may have been somewhat diminished in today's environment, future technological developments could have significant implications for hospitals, physicians, and other providers. Most hospitals did not anticipate the impact that technological advances in surgical techniques would have on the inpatient/outpatient mix of services; those that did gained a competitive advantage. Physicians, more than anyone, need to anticipate how these developments will affect the demands of their patients. Ophthalmic surgeons are now experiencing a jump in demand for radial keratomy by their near-sighted patients. Those who do not react to this demand may find that they have permanently lost patients to colleagues.

Understand the market area. Understanding a health care organization's market area provides the framework for all subsequent marketing. The first thing to do is delineate the current market area of the hospital or physician group. The method may vary with the type of service involved. The market area may be based on the residence of existing customers, distance parameters, or an area for which data are readily available, such as a county or zip code. For many services, it may be important to identify the primary, secondary, and even tertiary market areas. The extent to which customers (and prospective customers) are clustered or dispersed will be a factor here.

In some situations, the existing market area may not coincide with the objectives of the organization with regard to the particular service. The composition of the market area may be changing, making the characteristics of the resident consumers different. Or the organization's clientele may have "moved away" from the facility, as in the case of an inner-city, church-affiliated hospital whose patients have moved to the suburbs but continue to patronize the facility. The question to ask is: is this the market area I want to use as a framework for marketing?

Once a satisfactory market area has been delineated, the next step is to determine the present and future characteristics of its population. From a marketing perspective, this involves implementing a market audit, including an analysis of demographic trends (especially changes in population composition), socioeconomic trends, and psychographic characteristics. Relevant fertility, mortality, and migration trends should be identified. More to the point, the audit includes an analysis of trends in health services use and patterns of care. It is important to determine present and future demand for both inpatient and outpatient services, specific to the service in question and at the lowest level of geography possible. This market audit should also include an analysis of the population's ability to pay, combining socioeconomic information with insurance data. Projecting trends into the future is important, since few health services can be introduced overnight. Many require a two- or three-year startup period, so the characteristics of the population today are not nearly as important as their characteristics tomorrow.

Depending on the service, the market audit may include an inventory of existing providers. To the extent possible, the weaknesses of competitors should be determined. This becomes important later in making a realistic assessment of the capturable market.

Determine the level of need.   With an understanding of the market area, the marketer can focus on specific needs of the population for the service in question. Analyzing use trends in the market audit should provide the framework for identifying these needs.

It may be possible to identify the level of need for a service with some precision. For example, the number of annual births for a specific geographic area may be readily available to someone considering an obstetrics-related program. In most cases, however, actual data will not be available, and estimates of need will have to be made. Fortunately, a number of models have been developed to estimate and project the demand for a particular service. These modeling techniques require an understanding of the service area, and the more detailed the understanding, the better. Modeled data are not as good as actual data, but they are adequate. In any case, modeled data *must* be used if the level of need is being projected into the future.

Typically, the level of need is expressed as a percentage of the population (e.g., 20 percent of the adult population is affected by a clinically identifiable emotional condition) or a rate (e.g., the crude birth rate). The most common measures of need are prevalence and incidence rates used by epidemiologists and public health officials, and they provide the baseline data on which the rest of the analysis rests.

Estimate potential cases.   Once the level of need has been identified for the delineated market area, it is possible to specify the number of potential cases. A high prevalence rate by itself does not assure a meaningful market. Health care is a numbers game, and it takes a certain number of bodies to support any service. The population projections carried out above become important here, and their accuracy becomes an issue. If the level of need has been determined and adequate population figures are available, estimating potential cases is easy.

The key word here is "potential." Remember, one of the quirks of health care is that there is not a one-to-one match between those who need services and those who want them. In fact, the market is composed of those who need services and want them, those who need services and do not want them (or cannot or do not obtain them for some reason), those who do not truly need the services but want them, and those who neither need nor want the services. (The diagram below illustrates the possible combinations of needs, wants, and consumption.)

✔ Wants vs Needs

The Interface of Need and Want for Health Care Consumers

POSSIBLE CONSUMER SEGMENTS

1 – *Need services, but do not want or consume them*

2 – *Need and want services, but do not consume them*

3 – *Want services, but do not need or consume them*

4 – *Want, need, and consume services*

5 – *Need and consume services, but do not want them*

6 – *Want and consume services, but do not need them*

7 – *Consume services, but do not need or want them*

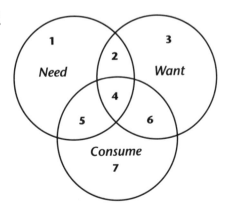

▲ **ORIENTATION TO HEALTH SERVICES**

Determine the distribution of cases.   Assuming that the market is of adequate size, another consideration is the distribution of cases within the service area. The importance of the case distribution varies with the type of service and the characteristics of the population. Some services require a concentrated population; others can serve a more dispersed market. Some services are supported by a local population and others by a more dispersed population. At the same time, some populations are more mobile than others or are otherwise more or less distance sensitive. Factors such as the type of service, the complexity of the problem, and even the level of patient affluence will influence the importance of location in the decision-making process.

Determine level of interest.   Since the level of need within the target population may not correspond with the level of interest, it is important to determine the extent to which the population really *wants* the service. This is the first point in the process that may require primary research. Ideally, no new program or service should be introduced without a consumer survey. The newer the service or the more unfamiliar the market, the greater the need. Untold numbers of programs have been unsuccessful because the actual level of interest of the target population was much less in reality than it was on paper.

Determining interest may be relatively straightforward. Surveys often ask consumers about their interest in the availability of a service and their willingness to use it if available. Marketers in health care found out early on, though, that these responses have to be carefully qualified. Typically, respondents express an interest in any new service that appears to benefit them or the community in general. However, when their use of the service is qualified by introducing locational or price factors, the level of interest may change. For example, one survey found that many consumers in a target area were interested in a hospital-sponsored fitness program. When the likely location was disclosed, interest waned. It waned even further when the proposed fee schedule was introduced.

HEALTH CARE

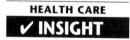

Consumers may approve of a service in theory, but not in practice—or location or price.

The more elective the service, the more important these qualifiers become.

Determine ability to pay. An increasingly important factor in health care marketing is the consumer's ability to pay. It is necessary to determine the potential payer mix of the target population and estimate the level of reimbursement expected for a particular service. Given the fact that different payers (e.g., commercial insurance, Medicare) offer different levels of reimbursement, the payer mix determines the actual level of payment. Obviously, the best coverage involves employer-sponsored commercial insurance. Other forms of private insurance (e.g., Blue Cross) are also desirable. While payments under Medicare and Medicaid are essentially guaranteed, the reimbursement rate tends to be less than that of commercial insurance.

Adjust for competition. Another critical step in the market assessment process is determining the level of competition. The extent that the market share can be decided for each significant competitor determines the understanding of the market potential. It is also necessary to assess the quality of the competition and its strengths and weaknesses in this market area vis-à-vis the proposed service. Competitive data are often hard to obtain, and the more specific the service, the greater challenge this may be. Estimates often have to be made, and it becomes important to be conservative in estimating the capturable market share.

Calculate cost/benefits. The next step is to calculate likely costs and benefits in introducing the service. Information on market potential, possible pricing structure, vulnerability of the competition, payment potential, and so forth have to be taken into consideration in determining whether or not to initiate the service and, if initiated, at what level. Numerous techniques are available for conducting cost-benefit analyses, and they will not be discussed here.

Once these steps have been carried out and the decision to initiate the program has been made, a marketing strategy must be formulated. Developing marketing plans is not an objective of this book, and marketers have access to abundant material on this topic. Refer to the suggested reading list and appendix for more information. The sections below do, however, discuss some of the elements found in a marketing plan.

Reaching the Health Care Consumer

Ways to reach the health care consumer are discussed in some detail in chapter eight, so they will not be belabored here. What is appropriate here is a presentation of possible frameworks that might be used for reaching the health care consumer. Remember, decision making in health care is a complex process that involves many players. As a result, a variety of frameworks are necessary. One involves marketing directly to consumers. Another deals with those entities that channel patients into health care, and this can be subdivided into a number of different approaches.

Marketing Directly to the Patient.   When one thinks of health care marketing, the first thing that comes to mind is taking the message directly to the end consumer, or the patient. This approach, incidentally, like the others, assumes that overall goals have been set, objectives have been established, and a general strategy has been formulated. The approach taken depends to a certain extent on whether the target is existing patients (customers) or potential patients (consumers). For existing patients, a variety of strategies are available. The primary objectives with this target audience include assuring that they are happy with the services they currently receive and that they are using all the services that are appropriate. With regard to the latter, the objective is not only that they consume appropriate services, but that they consume your services and not a competitor's.

Determining patients' level of satisfaction should be automatic when a practice or hospital profiles its existing patients. Contrary to the thinking of providers who do not want to give patients an opportunity to vent their frustrations, this information-gathering stage should be seen as a positive activity. The provider is gaining the opportunity to identify steps that can be taken to increase the satisfaction level of patients and ultimately keep them as loyal supporters.

The provider should also remember that patients typically do not change providers (or sue them!) unless they are dissatisfied with some aspect of the practice *not* related to the quality of care. Malpractice suits are typically triggered by a communication failure rather than by a negligent act itself. Patients who are happy with the relationship seldom sue their physicians even when negligence may be involved. Patients' complaints are usually easily resolved with a minimum of effort or change.

HEALTH CARE

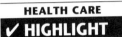 **HIGHLIGHT**

The customer satisfaction assessment offers another excellent opportunity. It lets the provider determine what the patient really wants. If a survey is appropriately structured, the provider can find out if there are additional services patients want, if another location would be more convenient for them, and other information that can help structure services to meet the needs of

As of 1990, 23 percent of people working in medium or large private firms had access to wellness programs as part of their benefit package.

the customer. Of course, the whims of the customer should not dictate the direction the service takes, but many of these suggestions can mean additional revenue for the provider. For example, with the fitness trend of the 1980s, consumers began demanding tests and regimens not typically offered by physicians or hospitals, such as wellness programs, stress tests, and nutritional counseling. Providers who picked up on this trend were able to position themselves as fitness-oriented providers and cash in on the numerous diagnostic tests requested.

Keeping existing patients happy can be summarized in one word—service. Health care providers are learning that health care consumers want the same level of service they have become accustomed to in other industries. They are no longer willing to wait for hours in the reception area, be treated curtly by office staff, or be cut off by the physician when trying to question a diagnosis or treatment. The success of many innovative forms of care (e.g., minor emergency centers) can be attributed to service.

The other objective for existing patients is making sure they consume all appropriate services and that they buy them from you. Health care providers have not been as aggressive in repeat sales and cross-selling as service providers in other industries. Hospitals and physicians often offer services that their existing customers are unaware of. Because of the lack of knowledge historically characterizing the health care consumer, the market has not been very organized. Hospital patients often do not realize that they can obtain a number of outpatient services from the same hospital or that the hospital may be affiliated with a nursing home, home health agency, or other needed health care organization.

Similarly, a practitioner may offer a variety of services that even long-time patients may be unaware of. After all, how does a patient find out these things? There is usually no formal means. Long-term patients may be going to someone else (even a competitor) for services that the practice offers. It may be something as simple as a senior citizen going to the health fair for an influenza shot or a mother taking her child to the health department for a school immunization when they would rather go to their regular physician if they were aware these services were offered.

Communication, then, becomes an important part of the service provided to existing patients. Active patients should be given as much useful information as possible while at the physician's office. Patients want to know about their health and the services that are available. This is a "teachable moment" that should not be missed. Since most patients are not regular users of the clinic or hospital, they should be contacted between visits by means of newsletters or other materials. Progressive practices have established "tickler files" that indicate when a patient is due for a checkup, when a patient's child is reaching school age, or other events that represent opportunities to provide information to patients and encourage use of the organization's services. As health facilities have become computerized, the opportunities for database marketing have increased. By maintaining a database of existing patients, it becomes possible to track their utilization patterns and develop strategies for repeat selling and cross-selling.

Consumers who are not already among the clientele of the health care organization obviously cannot be so readily assessed. However, to the extent that consumer information is available, efforts should be made to take the pulse of the marketplace. The approach here, of course, is not to cultivate customers (since you do not have them yet); it is one of awareness building. The provider needs to make people aware of the services offered, the quality of the practice and its personnel, and any advantages related to the organization (e.g., location, office hours, special services). The broader the range of services (e.g., those of a general hospital), the broader the marketing approach is likely to be. However, increasingly narrow audiences are being targeted. Even the mega-hospitals offering comprehensive services have come to realize that they cannot be all things to all people. Like the brand leaders in other industries, they are finding that niche players are eroding their market shares.

The other side of this coin involves developing new services or practice characteristics in keeping with the needs of the consumer. Some of these needs can be anticipated by keeping a pulse on the market and on societal trends. Some can be gleaned from market research involving consumer surveys or focus groups. No matter where the information comes from, a critical marketing objective should be to tailor services and practice characteristics to the needs of the consumer. This may mean offering new tests or procedures, opening a satellite office, or changing or expanding office hours. In some cases, the changing marketplace may offer a significant challenge. Hospitals that have not had a consumer orientation require a significant modification of mindset. Physician practices that have not emphasized prevention may find a marketplace demanding that type of orientation. Surgeons may find consumers demanding less invasive types of procedures.

Incidentally, it is not appropriate to talk about marketing services, even health services, without paying homage to the four Ps of marketing. Although it has not always been true in the past, all of these are important in health care today. With the emphasis on service that has emerged in health care, some observers are now talking about a fifth P—performance. Consumers who

HEALTH CARE
✔ HIGHLIGHT

In developing marketing strategies for both existing and potential patients, the health care provider needs to consider five Ps of marketing:

- *product*
- *price*
- *place*
- *promotion*
- *performance.*

are already discriminating between hospitals and clinics for their products, their prices, their locations, and the marketing approach they take are also increasingly judging a provider on the basis of the service provided.

Health care, like other industries, is now entering the age of relationship marketing. Relationship marketing means treating the customer interface like a long-term partnership rather than a one-time sale. It may mean sacrificing some short-term profits for a long-term relationship. This approach demands an in-depth understanding of the needs of the consumer and the flexibility and willingness to respond to these needs. It also calls for the integration of marketing activities. Advertising, promotions, customer service, and other components of the marketing process cannot be isolated. They must be integrated to present a consistent and persistent image of the health care organization. It also means that everyone in the organization must be oriented toward relationship development, management, and enhancement.

Marketing to the Patient Indirectly. While much marketing is geared toward the end user of services, health care is complicated by the fact that other parties, sometimes even those outside of health care, have input into the decision-making and financial aspects of health care consumption. For many services, control is being taken out of the hands of patients and placed in the hands of health maintenance organizations, insurance companies, and employers. Even physicians are finding that others are usurping their power. These intermediaries between the patient and the provider are determining the types of services that are appropriate, the level of payment, and even the providers to be used. The power is clearly shifting to these corporate players in the health care arena.

Physicians, however, still make most health care decisions. Virtually every health care organization that provides services to patients must interface with physicians in one way or another. Hospitals rely on physicians for their patient admission; physicians rely on other physicians for their referrals; pharmaceutical companies rely on physicians to prescribe their products; and nursing homes, home health care programs, and rehab facilities rely on physicians for their customers.

The marketing approach physicians should use depends on the nature of the relationship. The approach hospitals use to develop medical staff is clearly different from the promotional orientation pharmaceutical companies employ. The bottom line here is the same as for patients. Marketing to physicians involves determining their needs and how your organization can meet those needs. Physicians more than any other component of health care operate through networks and established relationships.

Insurance companies, preferred-provider organizations, health maintenance organizations, and other financial structures are increasingly controlling the patient's consumption patterns. These organizations are obviously quite different from the end user in their orientation and needs. As noted earlier, they respond to a different set of hot buttons and require a special approach. They are interested in cost-effectiveness, efficiency, and positive outcomes. They do share with the individual consumer an interest in value, and they are in a position to demand it. Like the consumer, they are also sensitive to the four (or five) Ps of marketing, although they may place different priorities on the individual components. They are particularly concerned about the nature of the product and the pricing structure.

Health care providers must be aware of two aspects when dealing with these types of organizations. They must use business-to-business marketing techniques, and they must emphasize relationships. Even government bureaucracies such as the Health Care Financing Administration respond better to providers with whom they have a satisfactory relationship. Ultimately, the provider must convince these third-party payers and intermediaries that it meets their needs in terms of products, pricing, service, and whatever other concerns they have.

A final consideration in indirect marketing to patients is the employer. Major employers are major purchasers of health care, and they are playing an increasing role in the use of health services. Employers are characterized by many of the same traits as the third-party payers above, but are in many ways much closer to the end user. They are, after all, negotiating on behalf of their employees. They want to save money and patronize low-cost providers, but not at the expense of quality. They are increasingly concerned about locational issues, since the site of the clinic may mean the difference between an hour and a whole day lost from work. Employers do not want to be in the health care business, so they are looking for providers or other health care organizations that can take over this responsibility.

The considerations above provide the basis for the marketing techniques discussed in chapter eight. Regardless of the nature of the customer, health care marketers will require a variety of marketing techniques and approaches to address a variety of targets. The process of transforming consumers into customers is complex in health care and requires a multipronged but well-integrated strategy.

....
The New Health Care "Consumer"

A Proliferation of Consumers

In the health care consumerism movement of the 1970s and 1980s, patients took more responsibility for their own health. Consumers insisted on being better informed and having some input into their treatment. They became smarter buyers of health services, researching the characteristics of hospitals and physicians, comparison shopping, and publishing directories of health care services and price lists for medical care and insurance coverage.

In the past, the doctor made these decisions, controlling the provision of care. While the patient has received the treatment, the physician typically "ordered" it. Thus, physicians account for the majority of health care expenditures. However, as a result of the developments of the 1980s, the proportion of expenditures physicians control has decreased from an estimated 88 percent in the early 1980s to barely 70 percent by the end of the decade.

We now realize, with our newly broadened perception of what constitutes health care, that many health care decisions are made without the benefit of a physician. Admittedly, physicians are needed for *medical* decisions, but consumers are increasingly taking responsibility for *health care* decisions.

At the same time, while the patient will remain a key player in health care consumption, in some ways her choices are being limited. Insurance companies, for example, now encourage the insured to utilize (or not utilize) certain services and/or providers. These health plans are increasingly "steering" patients to certain hospitals, physicians, and other providers. Steering has become so commonplace that many patients and patient advocates are complaining about the resulting restrictions on their freedom of choice.

In view of these developments, the real question for the decade is: Who will be the health care "customer" of the 1990s? Will the real customer be the party who is operated on, the party who makes the decisions about treatment, or the party who pays for the care?

Today, decision-making prerogative is being taken away from both the patient and the physician. Insurance companies, government insurance programs, and health maintenance organizations are taking on more of the decision-making responsibility. Rightly or wrongly, they are usurping the traditional prerogatives of medicine's vested interests.

Faced with increasing costs, insurers and other third-party payers began to more closely monitor the care being given and the charges levied. During the 1980s, they took the bold step of attempting to exert influence over the health care expenditure process. Not only did they do this by limiting their payments for certain services, but more importantly, they began to actually take on part of the decision-making responsibility. This included establishing preadmission screening criteria, performing concurrent monitoring of hospital patients to determine if appropriate (and cost-effective) medical protocols were being observed, and participating in the discharge planning process to assure that patients were discharged in a timely fashion and to the appropriate setting. When the Health Care Financing Administration (which operates the Medicare program) introduced its prospective payment system in the early 1980s, in effect it became a health care decision maker. This was a bold step that risked the animosity of physicians and hospitals alike.

Similarly, as employers have taken a more proactive role in financing health care, they too have taken on decision-making powers. They can do this most directly by attempting to influence the behavior of their employees. They might do this by offering incentives for healthy living and judicial use of the health care system. They might offer variations in insurance programs that encourage different types of behavior on the part of the insured. They may also negotiate with insurers, health maintenance organizations, and others who mediate between them and the providers of services. More and more, employers are negotiating directly with hospitals, physicians, and other providers to obtain the most favorable terms for themselves and their employees.

The entry of major employers into the process effectively completed the corporatization of health care. The individual customer (the patient) and the individual provider (the physician) have essentially been replaced by collective buyers and sellers. Today, corporate purchasers of care negotiate with corporate providers of care, often completely eliminating the input of both patients and physicians. Many argue that the incorporation of the health care system has been the major factor in its transformation and will determine its character in the 1990s.

Many would contend that the *real* customer in this environment is the one who pays the bill. In some cases, this is the patient. But in most cases, someone else is paying the bulk of the bill. Thus, one could consider the insurance company that is usually most at risk as the customer. Or is it the employer who, through company-sponsored insurance, ends up as the ultimate payer?

The real customer may not even be anyone directly involved in providing or financing care. Increasingly, health care policies are set in the political arena rather than the medical arena. Legislators at various levels of government are asked to address issues of inequity in the provision of services, adequate care for the medically indigent, appropriate levels of reimbursement, and the appropriateness of tax-exempt status for hospitals and other providers. To a certain extent, these too are "customers" with whom relationships need to be developed. Without the support of these policy-setting bodies, the health care system could face a political environment unfavorable to physicians, hospitals, and other providers.

Ultimately, the customer could be any of these—the one who actually receives the services, the one who decides the services are necessary, the one who pays the bill, or someone else. The answer depends, like many questions, on who is doing the asking. The fact of the matter is, the health care industry has many kinds of customers. The physician's customers include patients, as well as patients' families, other physicians (especially those who refer patients), the hospital with which he

The Corporatization of Health Care

CORPORATIZATION was one of the major developments to affect health care in the 1980s. That decade witnessed the demise of the individual player in health care and the emergence of the corporate player. The U.S. health care system had been built on trust—trust between doctor and patient, between doctor and doctor, and, to a lesser extent, between doctor and hospital. Medicine was considered a profession and, as such, relied on the integrity and qualities of the individuals involved.

By the beginning of the 1980s, hospitals were being transformed from community-service-oriented institutions into multipurpose organizations that often derived more profit from activities unrelated to patient care (e.g., food service, parking) than from the treatment of the sick. These organizations were combined into multihospital systems, many of them national in scope, and operated hospitals thousands of miles from corporate headquarters. Nursing homes were also combined into national chains. Physicians, dentists, and other health professionals obtained legal recognition as professional corporations, in many cases combining into large corporate practices.

Providers also took on other corporate characteristics. The individual relationships that had provided the basis for many transactions in the past were submerged by corporate boards that made decisions without considering the people involved. Many hospitals, nursing homes, and physician groups were taken over by professional managers, often with less background in health care than in the business world. As in other industries, health professionals saw control being shifted to the lawyers, accountants, and MBAs. The historical clinical orientation was replaced by an "administrative imperative."

While most would consider the corporatization of care pro-

▶

viders a natural development subsequent to the growth in size and complexity of the health care industry, few anticipated the extent to which the corporatization of care *purchasers* would occur during the late 1980s. The health maintenance organization movement that emerged in the 1970s was joined in the 1980s by preferred provider organizations, exclusive provider organizations, and other forms of managed care. These alternative delivery systems (actually alternative forms of financing) represented large groups of patients that to lesser or greater degrees served as bargaining agents for the "covered lives" enrolled in their programs. After all, their raison d'être was to control costs, and they were able to use their leverage to negotiate favorable terms with hospitals and other providers.

By the late 1980s, major employers emerged as active participants in the health care system. Spurred on by the seemingly uncontrollable increases in health care costs—of which employers were paying the lion's share—corporations began taking over the management of their employees.

The corporatization of health care has truly changed the manner in which business is conducted. The day of the individual patient interfacing with the individual physician is almost over. The patient who visits a clinic or enters a hospital is increasingly being "steered" to these providers by a managed-care program, an insurer, or an employer. We see groups of patients negotiating with groups of physicians or hospitals—i.e., corporations interfacing with other corporations.

For the health care marketer, this means that targeting individuals, while still a consideration, will become less important than targeting organizations. Similarly, the physician group must become an astute negotiator with managed-care programs and develop skills in capturing corporate accounts. Business-to-business marketing will replace much of the marketing now geared toward individual purchasers of care.

is affiliated, and the third-party payers he depends on for payment. The hospital also has a variety of customers—the patient, the patient's employer, the patient's insurer, the patient's doctor, and so forth.

By the late 1980s, another twist had been added as major purchasers of care (employers) took an active role in managing their employees' health care benefits. Arguing that they were ultimately responsible for the bill, they demanded input into the patient management process. They attempted to manage the spending process by controlling the sources of care available and by concurrently and retrospectively monitoring the use of services.

One consequence of these developments has been the emergence of "managed care" as a major factor in the medical management process. While traditional indemnity insurance is reactive, managed-care programs attempt to be proactive. They are designed to manage the illness process by having input on the front end, even prior to the occurrence of illness in some cases. In their most extreme forms, managed-care programs dictate the conditions under which various types of care can be provided, negotiate with specific providers of care for discount services, and indicate before the services are provided the amount they are willing to reimburse for a particular case.

These developments have had a significant impact on who controls the patient. By the end of the 1990s, an estimated 50 percent of health care consumers will be enrolled in managed-care programs. Another 20 percent will be covered under government insurance programs. This leaves 30 percent of the market for health care organizations to fight over, including the uninsured. The day of the walk-in patient is clearly over. Marketing must now be directed toward third-party payers, insurers, HMOs and PPOs, major employers, business coalitions, and even the managed-care brokers who have become the buyers (or at least the buyers' agents) for health care.

The Physician as Customer

During the 1980s, hospitals realized they had to become consumer-driven. However, many mistakenly believed that the patient was their primary customer. And many found out that the actual primary customer—the physician—did not appreciate being slighted. For a hospital, the physician is, or should be, its most important customer.

Most hospitals have been slow to recognize the importance of the physician in assuring a flow of patients. Hospitals that have held a monopoly in a community could perhaps justify a certain nonchalance with regard to a captive medical staff. After all, they were the only game in town. Eventually, hospitals with local competitors have begun to realize their life blood is the physician on the medical staff who admits patients.

The importance of physicians to hospitals goes beyond the simple admissions that generate daily room charges. Admitting physicians determine what tests are performed, what operations occur, what drugs are administered, and how long the patient remains hospitalized. The physician also determines whether a patient is referred to the hospital's skilled nursing facility, its rehabilitation facility, its nursing home, or its home health care program. These nonacute services are often profitable for the hospital but may be neglected when working with the medical staff to develop closer relationships.

Admitting physicians are not the only important ones. Hospitals must also cater to physicians who refer patients to the hospital's specialists. In fact, the greatest marketing challenge faced by many tertiary-care hospitals is to develop channels that will facilitate the referral of specialty patients from primary-care physicians in the area. If their specialists do not receive referrals, hospitals will see few admissions.

The hospital must determine what the physician as customer needs. Hospitals have had a difficult time determining to what incentives their physicians will respond. Communication between hospitals and their medical staffs has been surprisingly limited and often adversarial. This process is made more complicated by the fact that physicians associated with the hospital, either directly or through the referral network, can be segmented along a number of dimensions. Physicians have different needs depending on their specialties, whether they are office-based or hospital-based, whether they are solo or group practitioners, and the current stage of their careers.

The 1990s will clearly be a decade of bridge building between hospitals and their medical staffs. The age of medical staff development has finally arrived. Hospitals must develop systematic programs for developing relationships with all categories of physicians with whom they interface. This includes not only their heavy admitters, but those who refer to their admitters, their hospital-based support physicians (e.g., radiologists), and even residents in training. The need for these relationships has become even greater since the anticipated physician glut has not developed, and a growing shortage of physicians may be in the offing. Hospitals will have to develop relationships to hold on to the physicians they have already.

HEALTH CARE

✔ HIGHLIGHT

The projected number of new doctors needed in the next 15 years may range from 150,000 to 238,000, but the need for health technicians and other health-related workers will be much greater.

Hospitals have attempted to "market" to physicians in a variety of ways, although the process is not well-defined. Few hospitals have well-developed medical-staff development plans, so their attempts to market to physicians are often unsystematic and fragmented. The forms of marketing may be as simple as communication techniques such as newsletters and meetings. Some hospitals, however, have developed programs that place computer hookups in physician offices, subsidize equipment or office space, and provide various practice development services. An extreme example of physician marketing is the establishment of joint ventures with members of the medical staff as partners.

These attempts at "physician bonding" have had mixed results. The first rule of marketing is to determine what the customer really wants and needs. Hospitals seem to have made little progress in this regard and have had difficulty viewing issues from the physician's perspective. They have often made assumptions about physicians' needs and, rather than appearing to have the interests of these customers at heart, have come across as self-serving. Hospitals that hope to maintain loyal medical staffs during the 1990s will have to become more sophisticated marketers.

Hospitals are not the only entities that should be marketing to physicians. In fact, on a day-to-day basis, physicians themselves are more involved than hospitals (or at least should be) in marketing to physicians.

The Changing Role of America's Physicians

MORE SO than any other modern health care system, the U.S. system has been physician-centered. Since the emergence of scientific medicine in the early years of this century, the power of the physician has steadily increased. Spurred on by their "heroic" efforts in fighting the major health problems of the early 20th century, physicians were transformed from a status somewhere below used-car dealers to the lofty pinnacle they have enjoyed for many decades.

As the U.S. health care system rapidly expanded in the years following World War II, physicians began to play a larger and larger role. Medical doctors came to be recognized as the primary decision makers in the system. Only a physician could decide that a person was "sick," thus holding the ultimate power as gatekeeper.

The influence of the physician expanded so much that by the beginning of the 1980s, physicians controlled an estimated 75 to 80 percent of health care spending. Only a portion of this was actually spent for physician services, indicating the power that physicians exerted over other segments of the health care industry. The faith placed in physicians grew to the point that they were viewed as resources not only for solving medical problems, but for social, emotional, and spiritual problems as well. Patients placed tremendous trust in their physicians, and doctors ranked among the top in occupational prestige ratings. This prestige, of course, was reflected in their incomes, which have consistently been six or more times greater than the average worker. Aside from the significance of individual physicians, organized medicine became a powerful force in U.S. society, and the American Medical Association became the nation's major political lobbying group.

▶

The 1980s were a pivotal point in the progression of the medical profession. Faced with runaway medical costs, government agencies, insurers, and public-interest groups began looking for the causes of their financial woes. The gatekeeper role of the physician made him an obvious target. Physicians always ordered treatment for patients without regard to the cost and often without consideration of the clinical efficacy of the treatment. They often performed unnecessary tests and surgical procedures.

At the same time, physicians began getting adverse publicity related to other abuses such as Medicare fraud, self-referrals, and shady financial activities. While only a small proportion of physicians were involved, the entire profession became somewhat tainted. The number of malpractice suits multiplied, and juries awarded incredible sums for medical negligence. Malpractice premiums soared, causing many physicians to change their practice patterns and driving some out of the profession.

The publicized abuses caused a more sophisticated population to rethink the trust they had placed in their doctors. Public-opinion polls of the 1980s indicated a significant drop in the trust placed in physicians and a shift to a more realistic view of their capabilities. Patients who had been reluctant to say anything negative now freely expressed their opinions, even to physicians themselves. Formerly lifelong doctor-patient relationships were now freely dissolved, as patients sought doctors who would treat them like human beings and not gouge them financially.

Perhaps the biggest blow to the position of physicians came during the 1980s, when various third-party payers—the federal government, health maintenance organizations, and insurers—began to limit the control that physicians had in the patient management process. By the 1990s, a much smaller proportion of health services spendings was under physicians' control.

▶

The mid-to-late 1980s was a critical period for physicians. After an extended period of growth in patients, revenue, and prestige, they found that the patient pool was leveling off (partly due to an increase in physician supply), their incomes were leveling off and in some cases decreasing, and the respect they were used to receiving from patients and the general public was greatly diminished.

As a result, physicians have had to adapt or leave the profession. Many have limited their practices, taken early retirement, or moved into administrative or other nonclinical positions. The number of applicants to medical school dropped substantially in the 1980s, and teaching hospitals had difficulty filling positions in their residency training programs. Physicians have had to respond to changed conditions by becoming more consumer-oriented and placing an emphasis on service. Those who hope to prosper in the changed environment will have to combine strong business skills with clinical competence, customer service, and strong relationship development programs.

Hospital administrators or other staff have limited opportunities to interact with physicians. Yet physicians are in constant contact with other physicians. They may be accepting referrals from colleagues, sending patients to specialists, consulting on a colleague's case, "covering" for a colleague on hospital rounds or in the emergency room, or otherwise interacting with other physicians.

The more competitive environment will make the 1990s an era of physician-to-physician marketing. Physicians, more than anyone else in health care, have strong reservations about marketing. Yet most have been involved, often extensively, in informal marketing vis-à-vis their physician colleagues. It may not have taken the form of formal promotional material, but it has taken place in the doctors' lounge, through feedback on referrals, and on the golf course. At a time when the solo practitioner is disappearing, physicians depend more on one another for referrals, consultation, and counsel, even on nonmedical matters. Service-oriented physicians keep track of the referrals they receive and are conscientious about providing feedback and gratitude to referring physicians.

What most physicians really object to is not marketing, but advertising, although certain types of physicians have certainly been involved in advertising. To the extent that a physician or a physician group can promote itself without the perceived negative aspects of advertising, the 1990s will see an explosion of physician marketing activities.

Other groups are interested in marketing to physicians as well. Increasingly, third-party payers and major purchasers of care (such as employers) are attempting to enlist physicians in their service. Although group purchasers of care have done most of their negotiating with hospitals, these organizations are beginning to establish relationships with individual physicians. After all, hospitalization is a relatively rare occurrence; physician contact takes place quite often. Home health agencies, nursing homes, and suppliers of medical equipment and supplies also depend on physician referrals for much of their business.

One final group that should be mentioned because of its interest in physicians is the pharmaceutical industry. Manufacturers of therapeutic drugs depend on physicians to prescribe their drugs. As a result, the marketing activities directed toward physicians by pharmaceutical companies is a multibillion-dollar business. Pharmaceutical companies use a wide range of approaches in targeting their audience. These include advertising, direct mail, gifts, sponsorship of educational programs, trade-show exhibits, and direct sales. (Ironically, some pharmaceutical companies have been marketing directly to the patient, encouraging her through various media campaigns to request a particular drug from her physician.)

Insurers and Other Financers of Care

Just when marketers had gotten used to the idea of physicians as customers, they realized that the doctor's hands were being tied by the third-party payers that were beginning to call the shots. HMOs, PPOs, and even traditional insurers were actually attempting to influence the behavior of both providers and patients. Following the lead of the Medicare program, traditional insurers began to oversee the patient-management process. This is in stark contrast to their historical practice of essentially "rubber-stamping" bills submitted by hospitals and physicians. Both commercial insurers and the not-for-profit Blue Cross/ Blue Shield organizations began to monitor the treatment process and carefully scrutinize bills submitted for reimbursement under their programs.

The HMOs and PPOs set up as alternative delivery systems were actually established with the objective of controlling costs. From the beginning, their interest has been in controlling utilization and assuring that care was provided cost-effectively and efficiently. They oversee the providers under their control (physicians employed by an HMO) or with whom they have relationships. They are important customers to hospitals and physicians, not only because they control a large portion of the patient pool but because they dictate many of the terms of care and levels of reimbursement. Providers who do not have satisfactory relationships with these alternative delivery systems will have a difficult time surviving the 1990s.

Some managed-care organizations are not directly associated with a particular provider but link existing resources in the community to provide comprehensive services in a relatively controlled environment. Managed-care programs are attractive to employers and other major purchasers of care since they allow "one-stop" shopping for all health care needs. Further, the stated purpose of managed-care programs—to hold down the use and cost of care—attracts major purchasers who feel that hospitals, physicians, and other providers have a vested interest in the heavy use of health services.

The emergence of third-party payers, alternative delivery organizations, and managed-care programs has resulted in a partial shift in emphasis from consumer marketing to business-to-business marketing. Providers must develop mutually beneficial relationships with these third-party payers if they expect prompt, reasonable financial management.

Employers and Business Coalitions

Just when hospitals and other providers were getting comfortable with the influence of third-party payers, business coalitions and other major purchasers of care entered the picture. Formal groups of purchasers perhaps represent the end product of the incorporation of health care. Care providers have already become highly formalized—into hospital and nursing-home chains, ever-larger physician groups, and corporately sponsored alternative-care settings. Those involved in the financing of care—the insurers, HMOs, and others—have bureaucratized the financial side of health care. Now, employers and business coalitions have completed the circle by using their employees' combined buying power as leverage in negotiating with both providers and third-party payers.

During the 1970s, many industry observers offered progressive suggestions in the health care arena. Conventional wisdom, however, held that these ideas would never come to fruition because of the entrenched character of health care's vested interests. But many of these changes did occur, primarily because of the greater role employers took in managing health care. By the 1980s, this role had expanded dramatically, and major employers had been transformed from passive bankrollers to active players in the system. And by the early 1990s, representatives of big business were marching on Washington demanding some type of national health insurance program by the end of the decade!

HEALTH CARE

✔ INSIGHT

Only in the U.S. do employers foot the lion's share of health insurance costs.

The U.S. is the only developed society in which most health insurance is sponsored by and extensively subsidized by the private sector. As a result, U.S. businesses pay the largest share of the nation's health care bill. Not only is the bill large, it has been increasing much faster than other components of business expenses. The cost of health benefits adds a great deal to the cost of American products. Some argue that employer subsidization of health insurance has even put U.S. industry at a competitive disadvantage with foreign producers.

Not only do employers bear a large share of the costs, they also suffer the consequences of an inefficient system. It is one thing to pay fair prices for adequate care, but all too often employers have felt their health care benefit funds were spent on ineffective and inefficient care. The actual bill only begins to reflect the costs. Time off from work for employees who are not processed efficiently and repeat episodes for employees who were not properly cared for add to these costs. This situation became particularly noteworthy once employers began to offer coverage for psychological problems and substance abuse. They often found themselves with "revolving door" employees who the system could not seem to "cure."

As costs continued to rise during the 1980s, employers felt they were paying an increasingly disproportionate share of the nation's health care bill. At the same time, they realized that they actually controlled much of the consumption of health services. Health insurance benefits were previously seen as a cost of doing business: something put in place and then ignored. By the mid-1980s, this stance was no longer tenable, and employers realized that a proactive role was necessary. This situation encouraged employers to establish business coalitions to share information and provide a larger bargaining unit. With these coalitions, they could negotiate more aggressively with insurers and providers. This would also provide a means to influence the behavior of their employees.

The employer as health care consumer has added a new twist to health care marketing. As with the third-party payers, marketing to employers calls for a business-to-business marketing approach. Targeting a corporate customer is very different from targeting the individual consumer. It requires a different orientation, a different message, and a different marketing structure. For example, direct sales may not be an effective way to attract individual patients, but it is an essential approach in marketing to corporate customers.

Once meant to refer to the provision of services in the workplace related to on-the-job health and safety, "industrial health" now refers to targeting employers for a variety of health-related goods and services. Today, hospitals approach employers, seeking to contract for their hospital and industrial accident care; physician groups target them about handling their workman's compensation business; minor medical centers want to provide them with work-related physicals and manage their routine health needs; industrial health specialists offer drug tests, OSHA consultation, and hearing-loss screening; and health personnel agencies want to provide rent-a-nurse services.

Targeting employers for the sale of health services calls for different approaches than those taught in traditional marketing textbooks. Their "hot buttons" are likely to be quite different than those of the actual consumers of the services. The employer operates at a different level and, although generally concerned that employees be well treated personally, focuses on efficiency, effectiveness, and value. The prestige of the provider may not be important in the face of the practical need to return employees to the job quickly, inexpensively, and without relapses. Many employers, in fact, have sought out relationships with organizations that could guarantee these features.

New Constituents for Health Care Providers

In the 1980s, a whole new category of "customers" for health care providers emerged. These include the regulators, accreditors, policy setters, and decision makers. Many of these customers are actually outside of health care and operate in political, social, or economic spheres. As such, their agendas are likely to be different than those of the traditional wielders of power in health care. In fact, because of these new forces, marketers are getting fewer and fewer questions about market segments and more questions like: How can we justify eliminating this service? How can we demonstrate that we deserve our tax-exempt status? How can we demonstrate that we are an equal-opportunity organization?

These new constituents also include the press and public-interest groups, both of which serve as intermediaries between the public and the health care industry. The press has become increasingly critical of the health care system, and exposés of hospitals, physicians, insurers, and other health care entities have become common. The press actually reflects a growing negative sentiment on the part of the general public.

Public-interest groups have become more active in compiling information on health care providers and disseminating this information to the public. More importantly, they have been active in providing this information to policy setters and have become increasingly vocal in lobbying for legislation that would mandate a more consumer-sensitive health care system.

In the past, these types of customers have been handled with a public-relations approach, an approach that was probably sufficient at a time when hospitals and physicians were considered beyond reproach. A publicist could handle most issues with a glossover, and the controversy was soon forgotten. Today, however, a sophisticated marketing approach is required. Issues like the adequacy of charity care, discriminatory treatment practices, and tax-exempt status call for

> **HEALTH CARE**
> ✔ **INSIGHT**
>
> *Communicating with health care customers is a growing challenge, as the constellation of constituents diversifies.*

more than public relations. They demand a systematic approach, including careful research and well-developed marketing initiatives.

Responding to Customer Diversity

As health care enters the 1990s, health care providers and other health care organizations are faced with a different world. Virtually every health care organization—whether it is a hospital, a physician group, an HMO, or a medical-supply company—is likely to face a constellation of potential consumers. This proliferation calls for a diversification in marketing messages. Customers' sensitivity to issues varies widely. The general public may respond to certain cues, while existing customers may be sensitive to other issues. Similarly, unaffiliated physicians may have different "hot buttons" than physicians already on the medical staff. Insurers may respond to one set of issues, health maintenance organizations to another, and employers to yet another. The health care marketer of the 1990s must be truly versatile to meet this challenge.

This diversity of consumer groups, however, does have one factor in common: an insistence on relationship development. Whether marketing to individual consumers, physicians, insurers, or employers, the underlying theme must involve creating and maintaining relationships.

The movement toward more integrated care, more systematic care, and more continuous care—in fact, the entire managed-care movement—focuses on the establishment of working relationships that ensure not only continuity of patient care, but the ability to control and predict the flow of resources within the system. Chapter eight discusses relationship marketing in more detail.

....
Market Data in Health Care

Who *Are* These People?

The health care industry has been something of a paradox when it comes to data. While health care providers generate tons of data, until recently, they knew virtually nothing about their customers. At the facility level, health care providers have relied on data generated through routine administrative procedures related to admissions, surgical activity, and patient billing. These data were seldom collected in a format useful for market research or planning purposes. At the national level, health-related data were generated by a limited number of sources and were not widely accessible.

To anyone outside of health care, it may seem incredible that one of the largest industries in the economy had not developed adequate market data by the 1980s. Historically, though, there had been no need for market intelligence. Most health care providers had a local orientation, and health services were fragmented, making systematic data collection difficult. Much of the data, particularly on patients, was considered proprietary. Most hospitals, physicians, and other providers of care were reluctant to provide information on their operations to the public.

Federal agencies collected *some* data at the national level. Information on the use of health services was sometimes available, although it was seldom keyed to local geography. At the county and state levels, birth and death certificates provided data on such health-related issues as fertility and mortality. In some areas, limited data on health service use had also been collected. During periods when health planning was supported by the federal government, state and local health-planning agencies collected data related to a comprehensive array of health care issues. These activities took place primarily during the mid-1960s and mid-1970s but were essentially eliminated by the Reagan administration of the 1980s.

Although well intended, data collection efforts prior to the 1980s were relatively primitive, and the technology for managing and accessing these data easily was not available. Much of the information was collected from the perspective of government agencies and often did not coincide with realistic health-service geographic areas. Most important, however, was the fact that these data were not collected with marketing in mind. Since the health care system prior to the mid-1980s was not consumer-driven, little information was available on the knowledge, perceptions, needs, and use patterns of health care consumers.

Growing Demand for Health Consumer Data

Every development affecting health care during the 1980s resulted in an increased need for health care consumer data. The emerging interest in planning and marketing, the introduction of competition, and the shift to a consumer orientation, among other factors, mandate access to adequate data on both patients and consumers in general. Hospitals and other providers need to lay out guidelines for future development that realistically allow them to adapt to the changing environment. They have to develop capabilities for analyzing their market areas and drawing meaningful conclusions about the external environment. They need to develop and implement marketing plans that allow them to maintain their current customers and identify and cultivate new ones. All of these activities require access to accurate, detailed, and current market data.

Most importantly, as providers become consumer-driven, they have to develop an understanding of both existing and potential patients. In the past, it was not unusual for a hospital administrator or physician to have little understanding of patients. As a result, misconceptions of patient characteristics were often widespread. In view of the competition that has emerged, it is necessary not only to know about existing patients but to have a reasonable understanding of other consumers in the market.

Health care organizations are also finding, as those in other industries had, that costs associated with wrong planning or marketing decisions are enormous. If patients and revenue are guaranteed, as they were in the past, there is no risk involved in decision making. Today, however, the costs of establishing a new medical facility, developing a new service, or even recruiting an additional physician for a group practice are of such a magnitude that there is no room for error. Many hospital systems are now finding that one inappropriately sited facility can drag down several others that are favorably located.

The market for health-related data has also expanded as a result of changing factors that drew other interests into the field. Entrepreneurs with nonclinical backgrounds entering the field represent a business perspective used to thinking in terms of market intelligence. Employers require information so they can assess the treatment of their employees and interface intelligently with insurers, health maintenance organizations, and other third-party payers.

The growth in demand for health-related data has also been spurred by various agencies, governmental and nongovernmental, involved in regulating, planning, monitoring, and other activities. These include state planning agencies, federal funding agencies (such as Medicare), state insurance agencies, and agencies involved in public health activities.

The various third-party payers are another major force in the demand for data. They are finding that their continued survival requires an in-depth understanding of health-services use patterns, health care needs, and the preferences of health care consumers. Traditional insurance carriers have been joined by health maintenance organizations, preferred provider organizations, and other managed-care entities in seeking out and using detailed health care consumer data. And the newest forces boosting the demand for health consumer data are the employer and business coalitions that are taking an active role in controlling health care use and spending.

Types of Health Consumer Data

Those involved in health services are finding that not only do they need more data, they need more detailed data. A good example of this is demographic data. At one time, it was sufficient to have access to overall population counts, perhaps refined a little by age, sex, and race data. Today, it would be unthinkable to use unverified population counts or to conduct an analysis without detailed compositional data. While refined age and sex data are essential, it is now necessary to have access to a wide variety of socioeconomic data, too. It is imperative to have detailed income information, as well as detailed insurance coverage data. Carrying this further, one has to understand the industrial structure of a market in order to estimate the type and extent of insurance coverage.

It has also become necessary to have a clear understanding of marital status, family structure, and household characteristics. These factors have significant implications for the demand for health services and use patterns. Furthermore, the level of insurance coverage is, to a great extent, related to household type. Continuing shifts in the nation's household structure will have a significant impact on both the use of health services and the ability to pay for health care.

Before examining the various categories of health consumer data useful in marketing, it may be worthwhile to distinguish between *customers* and *consumers*. As commonly used, the term "customers" refers to those with whom one is already doing business. An inpatient at a hospital or an active patient of a physician is a customer. "Consumers" include existing customers as well as potential customers. Some potential customers may not be currently using health services or may be using a competitor's.

Customer data are primarily internal data, in that health care organizations collect information on their existing patients or clients. Hospitals maintain records on their patients, as do physicians and other practitioners. Similarly, insurers may maintain data on their insured and employers on their employees. In the past, hospital databases have been established for administrative and clinical functions, not for research, planning, or marketing. Internal data typically have two characteristics important to this discussion: (1) they are seldom collected with marketing in mind, and (2) they are seldom available outside the organization that collects them. It has been a real challenge for hospitals to adapt their systems to generate meaningful customer data. As database marketing becomes more of a reality for hospitals and other health care providers, managing internal customer data (and the ability to interface them with external data) will become critical.

Consumer data are essentially external data and, for our purposes, relate to both the characteristics of individual consumers within the external environment and the aggregate characteristics of the market itself. Data on consumers (including existing customers) deal with a number of factors, such as level of need, existing patterns of use, awareness/attitudes/preferences, and ability to pay, and are typically collected using sample surveys.

A distinction also should be made between *actual* and *modeled* data. Actual data refer to statistics that are "reality based," having been obtained by means of a census (for market area data), from registries (patient records), or from sample surveys. The results of sample surveys are not technically actual data, since certain inferences are made, but they can usually be treated as actual data.

Modeled data are based on statistical calculations that apply assumed rates to a particular population. For example, detailed utilization rates are now available for hospital admissions at the national level, broken down by diagnosis and procedure. These rates are typically available by age, sex, and race, and may even be adjusted for region of residence or other characteristics. One can apply the national or regional rates to the population in a particular market area. To the extent that compositional information (e.g., age distribution) is available, detailed estimates and projections of use can be made. Marketers can use similar modeling procedures to estimate the demand for and use of a variety of health care services.

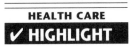

HEALTH CARE

✔ HIGHLIGHT

1990 hospital discharge rates by age, per 1,000:

<15 years	*43.9*
15-44	*101.7*
45-64	*133.1*
65 or older	*327.1*

Modeled data can serve as a useful proxy for actual data in many circumstances. Utilization rates for a particular service area are not likely to be available, so known rates from other areas can be used instead. The downside of modeled data rests with the assumptions that must be made. The basic assumption is that the behavior in the study area is similar to that of the "standard" population on which the utilization rates are based. The more detail that can be incorporated into the modeling process, the more likely the results are to approximate actual data.

Marketers need to consider all of the following categories of health data in order to understand the health care consumer and develop marketing initiatives.

Patient Characteristics.   Health care providers and those assisting them in planning or marketing activities must start by understanding the characteristics of their own patients. A basic profile of existing patients includes demographic and socioeconomic characteristics, case mix (e.g., diagnoses, procedures), payer mix, and place of residence. It is also important to obtain information about referring doctors and other medical relationships if possible and to have information on the patients' level of satisfaction. With this information, one can evaluate the "quality" of the current patient population, determine which segments are more "desirable," and identify the categories of patients one would like to target.

Market Area Population.   The first step in developing external, or consumer, data involves an overview of the service area population. This, of course, assumes that a service area (current or prospective) has been delineated. The overview should include population size (and trends), population composition (demographics, socioeconomics, etc.), and such health-specific information as type and extent of insurance coverage. The market area profile should provide the basis for all subsequent planning and marketing activities. The information should be detailed enough to allow for the analysis of subpopulations at various levels of geography (e.g., zip code, census tract).

Extent of Need.   Having identified the population of the service area and its general characteristics, it is necessary to determine the level of health services needed within that population. Local sources can provide some of this information. For example, local and state health departments collect fertility and mortality data (including cause-of-death information). Consumer surveys provide other, more detailed data. Marketers can use these data to determine the prevalence of various types of conditions and, perhaps more important, the extent to which these needs are unmet. Other statistics can be generated through the modeling techniques discussed above.

Utilization Patterns.   It is important to identify the existing patterns of health services utilization for the service area population. Depending on the needs of the organization, this could involve the level of inpatient activity, frequency of physician (or dentist) visits, use of various facilities (hospitals, minor emergency centers), participation in various programs (weight loss, fitness centers), and even enrollment in various insurance or managed care programs. One has to determine both the level and the type of utilization and, if possible, develop this information for various subgroups. One should also review the use of various competing services.

Psychographic Characteristics.   It has become increasingly common to profile consumers by their psychographic characteristics. Psychographics, as discussed in the chapters on consumption patterns and segmentation, refers essentially to attitudes and lifestyles. Psychographic analysis can help determine the likely health priorities and behavior of a population subgroup. This is important because groups that are similar demographically may be different in their lifestyle-influenced health behavior. For example, one category of elderly consumers prefers the traditional general practitioner for its primary-care needs, while another prefers the more specialized internist. Once identified, psychographics can help predict a category's propensity to use a wide variety of services.

Existing Relationships.   Relationship development has become increasingly important in health care, and the first step involves identifying existing relationships that may influence or reflect health care consumption. The most significant of these relationships is the one between patients and physicians, and in most marketing projects, it is important to determine which consumers use which types of physicians.

Again, this should be done by type of consumer and locality. Similarly, existing relationships with hospitals and other facilities or practitioners should also be determined. Unfortunately, this area has the least amount of existing data in today's health care environment.

Attitudes and Preferences.   Recent research has revealed a wide variety of consumer attitudes and preferences about health services. Even when consumers have limited knowledge regarding the credentials of the medical staff, they are likely to have some perception of the quality of services, the fee structure, the efficiency of treatment, and the personability of a health care provider. While these attitudes may not be "accurate," they are real to the consumers. Similarly, consumers have fairly well-established preferences about the types of services they like to use. For example, those who prefer orthopedic surgeons for the treatment of back problems are different than those who prefer chiropractors. Even within provider categories, there are differences in preferences related to such diverse factors as religious affiliation of the provider, location, amenities, and perceptions of quality.

Source of Payment.   Unlike other consumer groups, health care consumers need to be profiled by their source or sources of payment. It is important to know whether they are more likely to pay for health services out-of-pocket, with commercial insurance, or through a government insurance program. This situation has been made more complicated by the entry of various types of managed-care programs into the health care financing arena. Today, the payer mix of a service area is one of the most important considerations in planning, and the payer mix of a particular provider's patients is probably one of the best measures of that provider's financial viability.

"Hot Buttons."   As noted earlier, it is important to determine the factors to which different subgroups of consumers are likely to respond. The target population may be interested in quality, value, convenience, speed, location, amenities, or any combination of these and other factors. Their "hot buttons" will, to a certain extent, determine their preferences and use patterns. This information is important for servicing existing patients and attracting new customers.

The Database Boom

The 1980s witnessed a virtual explosion in health care databases. Some involved existing data registries that had never been very accessible, such as the vital statistics registries of the National Center for Health Statistics (NCHS). Other databases were constructed from information that had not been systematically organized in the past, such as Medicare payer data. Still other databases were constructed from scratch, such as the facilities databases and large-scale surveys of health care consumers developed by commercial vendors.

Associations, usually statewide, that compile, manipulate, and redistribute hospital utilization data have helped hospitals gain a better understanding of their patients. Sponsored by state agencies, hospital associations, or private vendors, mechanisms have been established to pool utilization data from participating facilities. A hospital can submit its patient records (with patient confidentiality intact) to the central clearinghouse where its data are merged with those from other hospitals. It can then get its data back and make comparisons with its competitors' characteristics (although the actual identity of participating hospitals may be masked).

With the growing pressure for better information, certain federal agencies have stepped up their efforts to collect and disseminate health-related data. Although much of this emphasis sprang more from concerns about rising government costs than from a desire to understand the market, it has involved many spillover benefits. Agencies like the Health Care Financing Administration (HCFA) expanded their data collection activities during the 1980s. HCFA began disseminating data on patients in the Medicare program and increased its funding of research on use patterns.

The NCHS has also stepped up its data collection activities based on both its registries and the sample surveys it conducts. It has improved the quality and scope of the data collected and made it more accessible, affordable, and user friendly. Federally supported data collection efforts have been most extensive with regard to use patterns and financing issues, although some of the surveys also address issues such as level of need, consumer preferences, and consumer knowledge.

NCHS: The Census Bureau of Health Care

THE NATIONAL Center for Health Statistics (NCHS) is considered the Census Bureau of health care. As an agency within the U.S. Department of Health and Human Services, NCHS performs a number of invaluable functions related to data on health and health care. For over 30 years, the center has carried out data collection, analysis, and dissemination activities and has pioneered the development of methodologies for research on health issues. NCHS also coordinates the state centers responsible for health data collection at the state level.

The center is responsible for the compilation, analysis, and publication of vital statistics (births, deaths, abortions) for the U.S. It is the last word in fertility and mortality data and, in conjunction with the Centers for Disease Control, generates morbidity data. More importantly for health care consumers, it conducts surveys based on community samples and patient use of various types of health facilities.

Perhaps the center's most important survey is the National Health Interview Survey (NHIS), through which it collects annual data from approximately 50,000 households. The NHIS is the nation's primary source of data on the prevalence of health conditions, the level of injuries and disabilities of the population, and health services use. Other community-based surveys include the National Medical Care Utilization and Expenditures Survey and the National Health and Nutrition Examination Survey.

The National Ambulatory Medical Care Survey, recently developed by NCHS, has become the most important source of data on ambulatory care. Based on a sample of

▶

the records of approximately 2,500 physicians, this facility-based survey collects data on diagnoses, treatment and medications prescribed, and characteristics of both physicians and patients. Other important facility-based surveys include the National Hospital Discharge Survey and the National Nursing Home Survey.

The NCHS provides its information in printed reports (e.g., publications like *Health, United States* and *Vital and Health Statistics*), tapes, and diskettes. It also sponsors conferences and workshops on its databases and methodologies. For the health care marketer, the center serves as an invaluable resource, representing the nation's largest collection of data on health behavior.

The growing demand for health care data has also been met by an increase in the number of vendors that offer data services. By the mid-1980s, many data vendors were catering to the health care industry, and some actually specialized in health care. These vendors provide services ranging from simple population figures for broad market areas to sophisticated analyses of a variety of market factors for very small units of geography. Commercial data vendors have established new databases, developed computer software for modeling various health consumer processes, developed estimates and projections, and repackaged data from other sources such as the federal government in more useful formats. They have also been active in conducting consumer surveys geared toward planning and marketing issues. These deal with topics not typically covered by government-sponsored surveys such as consumer attitudes, perceptions, and motivations.

Database information is typically available in printed form or on tape or diskette. Federal government databases tend to be inexpensive and conveniently formatted. Those developed by state agencies vary widely in cost and accessibility. Databases developed by nongovernmental agencies such as the AMA vary in cost and format, as do those from commercial vendors, although they tend to be more expensive than government databases.

Finally, health care providers are now collecting and managing data on their customers and on consumers in general. Hospitals with research staffs have reformatted their internal data to profile existing patients. They are conducting survey research on their patients and on the general population. Many hospitals have had to completely revamp their information management systems to make their internal data meaningful for research, marketing, and planning purposes.

Data Collection Methods

There are basically four kinds of data collection related to health care consumers: censuses, sample surveys, registries, and "synthetic" calculations of population estimates and projections. Censuses, sample surveys, and registries are the traditional sources, and they have been used increasingly since the mid-1980s.

A **census** enumerates all residents in a particular area. Because of the total coverage involved, censuses are major undertakings. The magnitude of the census-taking process in the U.S. is such that a census of the national population is conducted only every ten years. The 1990 census conducted by the U.S. Census Bureau collected little data directly related to health care, although there were some questions about fertility patterns and work and mobility limitations. The main benefit of the census from a health care perspective is the detailed demographic data it collects and disseminates for very small units of geography. These data serve as a basis for the calculations of health-related data made by vendors and others generating health consumer data.

Sample surveys have become the most common way of collecting health consumer data. Sample surveys involve interviews with a statistically selected sample of the population. If the sample is representative of the total population, the findings can be generalized to the total universe (conceding a small margin of error). Sample surveys have advantages over censuses in that they can be administered more often and collect more detailed data.

Much of what we now know about the utilization patterns of health care consumers and their preferences and attitudes has come from sample surveys. During the 1980s, it became common for hospitals to conduct their own surveys or to contract with market research firms to conduct them. Initially, few firms with the expertise required for health care surveys existed, and few hospitals had the in-house research capabilities required. A number of firms emerged that specialized in health care market research.

Conducting survey research about health care consumers is different from researching consumers in other industries. The nature of the problems involved, the organization of the health care system, and the motivations of health care consumers all make the study of health care consumption patterns difficult. Unfortunately, many market researchers have failed to appreciate this fact, and the literature is full of unsubstantiated findings and erroneous interpretations from misguided research.

As noted above, sample surveys are conducted by a variety of parties representing a variety of interests. In the private sector, a number of consulting and market research firms and vendors conduct surveys. These vary in frequency, scope, and geographic coverage, and include at least two major (100,000+ households) regularly conducted surveys of health care consumers. Increasingly, health care providers are conducting their own primary research, usually on their own patient populations. Research insti-

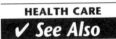

HEALTH CARE

✔ *See Also*

For more information on health care surveys, see the appendix on page 173.

tutes supported by universities or foundation or federal research funding also conduct sample surveys. NCHS, housed in the U.S. Department of Health and Human Services, conducts probably the most extensive array of sample surveys on the general public and administers similar surveys in a variety of health care settings (hospitals, nursing homes, and physician offices).

Registries or registration systems involve collecting, recording, and reporting data on a broad range of events, institutions, and individuals. Well-known registries include the Social Security

Can You Trust Health Care Consumer Surveys?

AS COMPETITION was introduced into health care, health care organizations required an in-depth understanding of consumer needs, preferences, and attitudes. Like other industries, health care turned to market surveys to obtain the information that had suddenly become so important.

Although some health care providers entered the business of market research themselves, most turned to existing firms for their market research needs. Few of these research organizations had previous experience in health care, but a significant industry soon developed to generate this information. Local market research firms began to conduct broad-based surveys of the American population's health care needs, preferences, and consumption patterns.

By the mid-1980s, the popular health care press was filled with findings from these research efforts. Every health care consultant felt compelled to produce periodic reports based on his or her primary research. Although this explosion in the availability of health consumer information was a positive development in an industry starved for data, many researchers were not experienced in health care. In their haste to publish, they often generated findings that were questionable due to sampling problems, data collection shortcomings, and/or other methodological difficulties.

At best, collecting data on health behavior is challenging. The nature of health care itself and the circumstances involved in the consumption of health services create problematic data collection. Health care behavior and beliefs can be more emotion-laden than perceptions and consumption patterns for other kinds of products and services. The fact that one's health (and perhaps one's life) is at stake limits the objectivity of re-

▶

sponses to health surveys. These is also a well-documented tendency for respondents to provide socially acceptable answers on such surveys.

It is particularly challenging to measure the perceptions and attitudes of health care consumers. Health care consumers are notoriously uninformed and are not likely to be able to speak authoritatively concerning most aspects of the health care industry, yet market researchers proceed as if consumers were well-informed, running the risk of basing strategic marketing decisions on consumer misinformation.

Even attempts at measuring use are not without their problems. Patients often have a poor understanding of the tests or treatments they have received and of the drugs prescribed for them. In fact, patients are so likely to forget about health services they have received that surveys requesting information for more than six months in the past are likely to be inaccurate. Surveys that ask patients to speculate on future health behavior are particularly problematic. Many people do not make health care decisions objectively, and they may have a limited time to make a decision.

Another factor detracting from the validity of health care consumer surveys is the discrepancy between what people say they will do and what they actually do. Thus, health care consumers often respond one way and behave another. In addition, researchers often make the mistake of determining the interest level in a particular service *without* indicating its location or price.

Do these drawbacks mean that all health care consumer research should be ignored? Not necessarily. Consumer research in health care should be evaluated like any other research. Marketers should be satisfied with the qualifications of the research organization, review the methodology, and find out exactly what questions were asked. Whatever approach is used, health care consumer research, like any other, should be taken with a grain of salt.

Administration's files, birth registries, and automobile licensing. To the extent that reporting is mandated, registries represent a comprehensive source of certain kinds of data.

The most useful registries for health care market data are those of "vital events"—i.e., births, deaths, and abortions. Other useful health-related registries include those on reportable diseases and AIDS maintained by the Centers for Disease Control. The Medicare "registry" has also become an important tool for monitoring the use of health services and the characteristics of users of certain types of services. Other health-related registries are less useful for consumer research but may be valuable for certain types of competitive analyses. These include the registries on physicians and other practitioners maintained by various state and national organizations. Information from these registries is becoming more accessible, and some such as Medicare make data available on computer tapes for easy access and analysis.

From Numbers to Solutions

In the past, health care organizations had a limited need for market data. When they did use them (e.g., for reporting purposes or site selection), they tended to use superficial data that were often of suspect quality. The questions of the day—the number of hospitals a population could support, the number of doctors that were required, or the level of services that were required—did not call for much more than basic population statistics.

By the mid-1980s, this situation had changed dramatically. Not only did the demand for data per se escalate, but higher standards of quality, detail, and accessibility were required. Detailed data on population trends and characteristics, levels of disease incidence, use patterns, and consumer behavior were now required. These data were needed for the market area, consumers in general, and the organization's existing customers.

Not only was there an emphasis on more and better data, but these data had to be turned into information. This meant being able to interpret the data and compare the statistics with other standards such as past performance and competitors. This need provided the impetus for the development of the commercial health data industry.

Ultimately, the need for information was transformed into a need for solutions. Health care decision makers need to convert the numbers into information and the information into answers to pressing planning and marketing problems. They need that "one number" that provides the solution to issues of site selection, new-service development, or marketing strategy. While some health care organizations have developed in-house capabilities for generating solutions, many have turned to outside consultants for assistance.

These heavier data demands would be impossible to meet if it were not for the much improved arsenal of weapons available to the health care marketer. The tools available for marketing research and planning just a few years ago seem relatively primitive by today's standards. Sophisticated market analysis capabilities have become increasingly common, with the ability to interface a variety of databases (both internal and external). If they cannot provide the complete solution, they can at least provide the guidance an analyst needs. Today, those involved in health care marketing and planning have access to large detailed datasets. Utilization rates can estimate the demand for both inpatient and outpatient services, as well as for special programs such as rehabilitation and substance abuse. Data vendors have developed applications that provide quick and efficient analysis of planning and marketing issues. With geocoding, for instance, marketers can better target both customers and potential consumers.

Much of this has been made possible, of course, by microcomputer technology and desktop analysis systems. With the speed and memory capabilities of microcomputers, sophisticated software systems can interface disparate databases and simultaneously analyze a variety of datasets.

The demand for health-related data shows no signs of abating. As the debate on national health insurance continues to heat up, there will be increasing interest in relevant health data. If some form of national health program is implemented, it is likely that more data on consumer behavior patterns will be required to monitor the system. For providers, the costs of mistakes will continue to rise assuring continued demand on their part.

During the 1990s, one can expect even better data availability and increased detail and quality. Ever more sophisticated models will be developed, and continued hardware and software development will add new capabilities to the arsenals of health care planners, marketers, and consultants. High-tech support such as satellite imaging will also contribute to the arsenal available for attacking marketing issues.

The appendix on page 173 lists a number of sources of health care consumer data. Although the list is not exhaustive (and sources of data come and go), it provides some indication of the available data.

CHAPTER EIGHT

Marketing Techniques for the 1990s

T HE TREATMENT OF CUSTOMERS by health care marketers is reminiscent of a comment made by Dr. William Masters (of Masters and Johnson fame) concerning the manner in which males had treated females sexually since World War II. He observed:

> Throughout the 1950s and 1960s, sex was something that men did *to* women. After the consciousness-raising developments of the 1960s, men starting doing sex *for* women. Finally, with the enlightenment of the 1970s and 1980s, men started having sex *with* women.

This is analogous to what has been happening in health care marketing. Marketers started out promoting *to* consumers as if they were simply sex objects to be seduced. Then they realized they were being insensitive to the needs of the consumer and began asking what they could do *for* customers. Now, marketers must determine what they can do *with* the customer, whether the customer is a patient, a physician, an HMO, or a business coalition.

Marketing Challenges of the 1990s

Of all tools available to health care providers, marketing programs can make the biggest, most direct, and longest-lasting contribution to profits. They can increase revenue by changing the payer mix, attracting new patients from targeted market segments, and emphasizing higher-profit services and procedures. Health care organizations have barely scratched the surface of the potential benefits of marketing.

Despite this tremendous potential, marketing in health care still faces an uphill battle in establishing its legitimacy. Having somehow survived the 1980s, health care marketing now finds itself facing even greater challenges. In fact, the 1990s are likely to be the make-it-or-break-it decade for health care marketing.

Although some unanticipated developments are likely (and there are some big unknowns, especially in the area of reimbursement), most of the trends that will affect health care marketing in the 1990s are already underway. The marketing techniques chosen for the 1990s must keep these trends in mind. The following factors will demand that health care marketers adopt a new marketing orientation.

More demanding consumers.   The patient/client/customer using health care services in the 1990s will be much more demanding than at any time in the past. This is true whether we are talking about individual patients, physician associates, or major employers. These groups now have more knowledge about health care, and with knowledge comes growing interest in playing a part in the process. Customers at all levels will demand accountability, cost-effectiveness, positive outcomes, and service. These customers will demand, above all, value. Consumers are already shopping around to evaluate service and price. Employers and business coalitions are also shopping for the best service and price. Third-party payers will not deal with health care providers who do not provide the value they expect.

Market heterogeneity and fragmentation.   The growing heterogeneity and fragmentation of the market will be a major challenge for marketers of the 1990s. Marketing approaches will have to be sensitive to the disparate needs and perspectives of widely diverse population segments. Not only will advertising copy have to be sensitive to the needs of various subgroups, the product, its packaging, the location of the service, and even office furnishings must be developed with these factors in mind.

Changing product mix.   Changing demographic characteristics, consumer preferences, technology, and even third-party reimbursement procedures mean an increasing demand for some services and shrinking demand for others. Coming into the 1990s, for example, there was a booming demand for obstetrical services; by the end of the decade, this demand will have dropped dramatically. Trends in consumer preferences must be anticipated to determine what services will experience increasing (or decreasing) demand. Technological advances could make some now unheard-of procedures commonplace. Decisions by third-party payers could dramatically alter demand patterns if, for example, they no longer covered open-heart surgery in favor of angioplasty or determined that preventive care should be emphasized.

Increasing cost of marketing mistakes. The costs involved in a wrong marketing decision have become astronomical. A poorly designed product, inappropriate packaging, the wrong message to the wrong audience, selecting the wrong site, providing the wrong services: these developments will be unacceptable in the 1990s. The costs of doing any of these things wrong are becoming prohibitive, and every aspect of marketing—from product to price to place to promotion—will have to be carefully thought out.

Factors in Choosing Marketing Techniques

The marketer must consider a number of factors in choosing which market techniques are most appropriate for the health care organization. These factors should be selected based on the overall goals of the organization. The issues discussed below provide guidance in choosing the appropriate marketing techniques.

Positioning the organization. The need to "position" the organization in the market cannot be overemphasized. As a marketing approach, positioning can take two forms. In the first, it refers to what the organization should be positioned *as.* Is the goal to have the organization seen as the clinic of the rich and famous, the low-cost provider, the prevention-oriented practice, the quality provider, or what? While a variety of marketing techniques can contribute to any of these goals, some will be more useful than others in view of a particular strategy.

In the second approach, the issue is what to position the organization *in relation to.* That is, does the hospital, clinic, or other provider want to position itself to capitalize on a growing affluent population, as the introducer of an innovative procedure, to benefit from shifts from an inpatient to an outpatient setting, or to take advantage of certain ready sources of referral? Again, the choices made will influence the type of marketing required. These positioning stances are quite different, and each requires a different approach.

Differentiating the organization.   At the same time an organization positions itself, and almost as a mandatory accompaniment, the organization must differentiate itself in the marketplace. Over the past decade, there has been a "democratization" of health care, as consumers better understand the system. Today's consumers know that most hospitals have some minimal level of quality, so they make their comparisons on the basis of other differentiating factors that are meaningful to them. In a community where one hospital is viewed as the provider for the affluent and another for the provider of the poor, there may be little difference in the quality of care provided. The difference is in the mind of the consumer. Differentiation depends in part on presenting a certain image. This may not be directly influenced by advertising, but if specialized services are offered or a particular niche is captured, the differentiation will take care of itself. Remember, perceptions are more important than reality; it is sometimes better to be differentiated in the consumer's mind than in actuality.

Product life cycle.   Like other products, health services can be viewed by life cycle. The life cycle aspect of health care may be a result of either changing technology or changing consumption patterns. For example, a certain trend may have run its course (e.g., psychotherapy) and reached the declining sector of its life cycle. Technological change, of course, is a well-recognized factor in product life cycles. As new technology is introduced, established procedures may go into decline while new procedures take off on a growth trajectory. Or changing demographic trends may portend that demand for a particular service has peaked, and another service, now in its growth stage, will replace it.

Aside from the obvious need to position the organization to capitalize on the most appropriate life-cycle stage, this process has important implications for health care marketing. There is a significant difference in marketing an innovative new service, taking advantage of booming growth for a newly popular service, and trying to maintain a reasonable share of a mature market where demand has stabilized. Each situation calls for a different marketing approach.

Cost-effectiveness.   A major consideration in choosing a marketing technique in today's market is its relative cost-effectiveness. In the early days of health care marketing, there was such a rush to get on the marketing bandwagon that cost was not a major factor. By the end of the decade, however, there was growing determination on the part of health care organizations to get the most bang for their buck. They evaluated traditional marketing techniques in this new light and, in many cases, were unable to verify their efficacy.

The nature of the customer.   Another consideration in choosing among marketing techniques is the nature of the customer. Some health services are offered on a one-shot basis; i.e., the provider is likely to see the patient one time, and every customer is a new customer. Other providers may see the same customer several times while providing the same service (e.g., for postoperative followup after surgery). Still other providers may see the same patient several times and provide a variety of services. The pattern of interaction will dictate the type of marketing used. Constantly attracting new customers requires one approach, keeping existing customers satisfied enough that they continue to return for treatment requires another, and making existing customers aware of the variety of services available requires yet another.

New Techniques for a New Environment

The 1980s were a period of transformation in health care and experimentation in health care marketing. The 1990s promise to be the decade in which some marketing techniques come to the fore and others are deemphasized. Some of the tried-and-proved techniques, in other industries at least, may fade into the background, while innovative approaches specific to health care may emerge. The sections below review a variety of marketing techniques and discuss their relevance for health care.

Traditional media campaigns.   What people think of as marketing will be quite different in the 1990s. For many people, and especially health professionals, marketing *is* advertising. Despite some reservations, many health care providers jumped into advertising in the 1980s. Hospitals led the way, but were joined by other organizations such as minor medical centers and freestanding diagnostic centers. Managed-care plans advertised in an attempt to attract industrial clients. Physicians resisted advertising initially, but many eventually came along. Chiropractors and certain other practitioners had fewer reservations and unabashedly began advertising.

Advertising in this sense focuses on the traditional mass media. These media include television, radio, newspapers, magazines, and outdoor (primarily billboards). They are called mass media because they tend to provide relatively untargeted exposure to the general public. These media have advantages and disadvantages, briefly described below.

Television has been seen as a glamour medium and is often the one that first comes to mind when an organization considers mass marketing for the first time. Television offers the opportunity to take a message into a large number of households, reaching into the millions if national advertising is considered. Television is expensive in both production costs and air time. Its major drawback, however, is its inefficiency. Except for highly targeted stations, television advertising represents a scattershot approach. Even with the information now available on viewing habits, the likelihood of hitting a specific target is low. In view of the situation for many health care providers today, reaching the right consumers is more important than reaching the most consumers. Furthermore, the competition for television exposure is incredible, and viewers are often unable to remember the sponsors of advertisements. After a torrid romance with television advertising, most health care providers, like many other industries, are withdrawing their television dollars and turning to more efficient methods.

Many view **radio** similarly to television. To a certain extent, it also represents a shotgun approach to advertising, although radio listeners are more segmented than television viewers. The cost of radio production and air time are considerably less than for television. Despite these advantages, the effective exposure time for radio "spots" is limited, and because of the commercial clutter involved, there is a tendency to tune out advertisements. Many health care providers continue to use radio advertising, however, even after pulling back from television advertising.

Newspapers were also seen initially as a potential channel for advertising health-related services. They appear to have many benefits as an advertising medium. They are easily accessible, not prohibitively expensive, and carry a certain aura of believability. On the other hand, they are virtually useless for targeting a particular market segment and, in fact, may be most often read by segments of the market that the advertiser would rather not serve. Although many health care providers still feel it is necessary to advertise in the local newspaper, the zeal for this method of advertising waned as we entered the 1990s.

Some health care advertisers have viewed **magazines** as an alternative to newspapers. Magazines have several advantages over newspapers in that they have a longer useful life and can produce higher-quality advertisements. More important, except for a few general-interest publications, most magazines have become relatively tightly targeted. But most health care providers serve a local market, and at that level, the availability of outlets for magazine advertising is limited. As with newspapers, there has also been some slippage in the perceived efficacy of magazine advertising.

The other form of traditional media advertising is generically referred to as **outdoor advertising** and typically refers to billboards. Some health care providers, managed-care programs, and other organizations have used billboards to get their messages across. While billboards are relatively inexpensive and have a repetition effect, they are probably not particularly useful for the message that most health care providers hope to convey. They have limited space for "copy," and it may be difficult to say what needs to be said. Even with careful placement of billboard ads, the ability to target selected groups is limited. The effectiveness of billboards is questionable, and many health care organizations consider it a form of advertising with which they do not want to be associated.

Media Advertising and Health Care

WHEN health care organizations turned to marketing, their typical first response was to use traditional media advertising. Hospitals in particular began advertising on television and radio, in newspapers and magazines, and on billboards. While some of these media are suited to the marketing needs of health care organizations, others are not. The table below indicates the pros and cons of various forms of media advertising for hospitals and other health care organizations.

MEDIUM	ADVANTAGES	DISADVANTAGES
Television	High attention level Implies quality organization Multisensory impact Potential high impact	Limited targeting ability (network) Overly specific targeting (cable) Short message life Excessive competition for attention High production/time costs Perceived extravagance
Radio	Low production/time costs Good targeting ability Local market orientation	Less impact than visuals Short message life Excessive competition for attention
Newspaper	Easily accessible Limited time commitment Believable Local market orientation	Limited targeting ability Short "shelf life" Low print quality
Magazines	Relatively long "shelf life" Good targeting ability Local/national options Can imply high quality	Long lead time required Possible visual clutter Potential poor placement
Billboards	Repeat exposure Low cost Visual impact	Limited targeting ability Limited message Could imply low quality

The traditional media campaign is a candidate for the endangered-species list. This form of advertising is roundly criticized for being expensive (or at least not delivering very much bang for the buck) and having limited ability to target specific populations. As in other industries, many health care organizations are rethinking their marketing mix and advertising budgets. Once these activities are carefully considered, more often than not the decision is to reduce spending on traditional media.

One aspect of media advertising that has become increasingly popular is the "advertorial." Whether presented as a newspaper ad or a radio spot, the advertorial serves the advertising needs of the organization, but in a manner that presents it as concerned about things other than attracting patients. Some advertorials can actually be run as public service announcements, thereby increasing the benefit to the health care organization.

Public relations.   In the past, health care providers have used public relations as their major interface with the public. It was a component of hospital operations long before the concept of marketing was formally accepted. Public relations typically involve interface with the media (particularly newspapers), support for various community programs, image enhancement, and some of the outreach activities discussed below. This activity has come to involve government relations and even some interface with managed-care programs, employers, and other purchasers of care as the incorporation of the purchase of care has picked up steam.

As a form of marketing, public relations typically functioned independently of market research and was often seen as a way to gloss over the problems of an organization and hype its strengths. Public relations personnel were not usually trained marketers and actually experienced some conflict with marketers once the latter were brought on board. These spokespeople's activities are still important for the health care organization, although it appears that the world has become too sophisticated for what used to be considered public relations. Marketing has assumed some of these functions, and some hospitals have set up government-relations offices from which individuals with more specialized skills interface with government agencies. Also, many public relations functions have become part of community outreach activities described below.

Community outreach. During the 1980s, community outreach activities became increasingly popular among hospitals, physicians, and other care providers. A variety of activities are included under this heading, such as health fairs, sponsorship of community health-related events, provision of free services to underserved populations, and media appearances. Media appearances differ from the traditional public relations press release in that expert spokespeople for the organization appear on radio or television to offer substantive information about the services provided, rather than the superficial message presented by public relations personnel.

It has been difficult to gauge the effectiveness of some of the programs that fall under the heading of community outreach. Perhaps health fairs have been praised the most for their ability to garner local exposure for the organization or program. The fact that exposure occurs is unquestionable; many health care providers contend that they identify many unmet health needs among health fair patrons, many of whom can be converted into customers. On the other hand, those who attend health fairs presumably to obtain the free services may not be the types of customers some health care organizations are attempting to attract.

Direct marketing. Direct marketing is being hailed as the new wave of health care marketing, and it is beginning to replace much of the traditional media as a means of reaching select customers. Direct marketing involves a number of discrete activities that have in common the fact that they market directly to the consumer without the intermediary of television, radio, or some other medium. Direct marketing includes direct sales, direct mail, and telemarketing, all of which are designed to carry a personalized message straight to the customer or prospective customer with maximum efficiency. With direct marketing, marketers can fairly precisely target audiences for a particular service, overcoming the shotgun tendency of the mass media. At the same time, direct marketing addresses the cost issue by providing more bang for the buck, and it addresses the effectiveness issue in that its benefits are much easier to track.

Direct mail is being increasingly used by many industries, and its advantages are now recognized by health care organizations. With the technology now available, it is possible to identify, even down to the household level, prospective users of a particular service. This same technology allows health care organizations to know enough about consumers to package products and tailor messages responsive to their hot buttons. Furthermore, it allows the provider to avoid subpopulations that it doesn't want to target.

Direct mail can expose targeted populations to repeat messages or sequenced messages to create a desired effect. Direct-mail campaigns can also be coordinated with other marketing activities. If properly executed, direct-mail campaigns are highly cost-effective, and their financial benefit can generally be determined.

The disadvantages of direct-mail campaigns mostly reflect the medium used. Consumers are swamped with "junk" mail, and it may be difficult to get the target's attention. It usually works best if the target has already been a patient, and there is some "hook" to attract his attention. Some consumers object to being solicited by hospitals or other providers by mail, and the reaction is likely to vary with the target audience. A misdirected direct-mail campaign could end up costing much more than it is worth. For organizations targeting physicians, direct mail seems like a reasonable way to get the message into the physician's hands. But in view of the amount of mail received by the typical physician (and the fact that someone else may screen the mail), it might be wise to consider another approach.

HEALTH CARE

✔ INSIGHT

Poor direct marketing to busy doctors may be worse than none at all.

Telemarketing is another form of direct marketing that health care organizations are finding useful, even though one gets the impression that there is more talk than action so far. Many health professionals have become convinced that the benefits of telemarketing demonstrated in other industries are transferable to health care. One side of the telemarketing coin involves incoming calls. Health care organizations can set up centers, with toll-free numbers if appropriate, that can

Direct Mail Applications in Health Care

UNTIL THE late 1980s, few health care providers considered direct mail a viable form of marketing. Hospital administrators in particular felt that illness episodes were unpredictable and that the choice of provider was typically controlled by someone other than the patient. While it may have been possible to improve the institution's image through advertising, it was not feasible to influence the behavior of individual patients.

This perspective, of course, reflects the inpatient orientation so prevalent among hospital administrators. After all, direct solicitations aimed at individual patients—regardless of the quantity or quality—were not likely to have much impact if the targeted patients did not need the services or if someone else was making the decision about health-services use.

Progressive health care organizations have moved beyond this mindset. Shifts from acute to chronic conditions and from the inpatient to the outpatient setting have placed more control in the hands of patients themselves. The increase in elective surgery has contributed to the patient's decision-making role. Marketing-oriented hospitals and physicians realize that patients do make decisions, and it is their responsibility to take advantage of these opportunities by marketing to patients and prospective patients accordingly.

This situation makes direct mail a much more attractive alternative for marketing activities. To the extent that certain population segments should be targeted for certain services, direct mail is the only reasonable alternative to traditional media campaigns. With direct mail, the hospital or other provider can control which households it solicits for a particular service. Not every household is a candidate for a fitness program, so it becomes important to identify and contact those

▶

that are. At the same time, the provider may *not* want to attract certain population segments for certain services, and direct marketing offers this avoidance option, too.

With direct-mail campaigns, providers can also control the timing of the marketing initiative. To the extent that various health care events are "sequenced," it is necessary to time marketing efforts carefully. This is much more difficult to accomplish with media advertising than it is with direct mail. If a woman delivers a baby at a hospital, it may be desirable to encourage her to use pediatric services at that hospital. It is clearly more expedient to do this via direct mail than through television or newspapers.

Although some organizations consider direct mail an invasion of privacy and a contribution to the junk-mail flood that people find so offensive, many providers realize that properly executed campaigns can actually enhance an organization's image. Physicians who would never consider "advertising" are willing to send out letters to their patients announcing a new service or reminding them of a scheduled visit.

While direct-mail campaigns are not cheap, they are inexpensive compared with most other forms of media. Hundreds of prime prospects can be solicited directly and relatively personally several times for the price of a single mass-media advertisement. As a result, some health care organizations are shifting marketing dollars from media advertising to direct-mail programs. Hospitals are using direct mail to increase penetration for existing services, introduce new services, provide information on the programs and professionals available, and generally maintain communications with customers and prospective customers. Some hospitals even use direct mail to solicit contributions for fund-raising drives.

process calls from a variety of categories of consumers and, hopefully, turn them into customers. These services could include ask-a-nurse services, physician referral services, insurance (including Medicare) hot lines, and centers that respond to specific promotions. The better-designed incoming telemarketing programs can direct these callers to resources that may result in followup "sales." They also have the advantage of creating a database of those inquiring into hospital programs.

Other telemarketing programs for incoming calls include physician-consultation services and employer-information services (e.g., for industrial-health programs). Physician consultation lines attempt to shore up weaknesses in referral networks. They have been relatively successful, but they have to be well run or a potentially positive experience could turn into a public relations *faux pas.*

Outgoing telemarketing programs have been less developed, and hospitals and other providers are understandably resistant to being too aggressive. Marketers are probably more sold on the benefits of this marketing approach than are hospital administrators. Although "cold calls" on potential health care customers may be controversial, followup calls and cross-selling efforts directed at existing patients are more widely accepted. Physicians and dentists who make appointment reminder and visit followup telephone calls are doing low-level telemarketing that is seen in a positive light. Patient satisfaction surveys could also be placed in this category, and they can serve as a mechanism for testing new ideas and introducing new services.

Telemarketing requires a considerable amount of effort, and the costs involved in maintaining either incoming or outgoing service are not small. Telemarketing services must be carefully planned and designed. In addition, they must be constantly monitored, or the potential benefits become diluted. They can be controversial and must be handled very diplomatically. Users have unlimited horror stories of calling to cross-sell to a previous hospital patient without realizing that the patient had died *in their hospital,* or loyal physicians finding out that competitors who do not even admit to a hospital are listed along with them on the physician-referral service.

The incorporation of health care on both the buyer and seller sides has prompted health care organizations to get into **direct sales**.

Direct sales are nothing new to pharmaceutical companies and medical supply companies that rely on a sales force to personally get their message out to prospective customers. For hospitals and other providers of care, the notion of sending "salesmen" out into the field has been hard to swallow. Nevertheless, as the focus shifts from catering to the individual patient to soliciting wholesale business from major-care purchasers, they are finding the prospect of a sales force more palatable.

Hospitals have developed sales forces to call on industry, business coalitions, alternative-delivery systems, insurers, and physicians. While the specific objectives of these sales representatives vary, their main purpose is relationship development. Hospital representatives may be sent out to sell an industrial health program to a local employer, to convince members of the business coalition of the advantages of affiliating with the hospital, to establish relationships with managed-care programs, and so forth. They may be sent out to physicians to attract nonadmitters to the hospital, troubleshoot for existing medical staff members, and otherwise establish and maintain relationships with physicians and customers. Representatives of special-care programs such as rehabilitation or substance-abuse facilities are calling on the same types of organizations in an effort to attract their business. Physician groups are also beginning to see the usefulness of direct sales; some have personnel who contact referring physicians or potential customers for industrial-health programs.

Despite the initial apprehension on the part of health care providers, most are finding that some form of sales force is necessary to maintain any sort of market position. After all, decisions are increasingly made by organizations rather than individuals, and direct sales is a good way to contact such organizations.

As with telemarketing, developing direct-sales capability requires considerable effort and expense. This marketing component requires constant monitoring and finetuning as it progresses. Also, like telemarketing, direct sales is controversial and has tremendous potential for disaster. Representatives in the field can be a liability, and one bad impression could be a deal killer. Another important consideration, and a problem often faced by hospitals, involves sending sales representatives into the field when they actually have nothing to sell. Some hospitals may call on physicians to help meet their needs, only to find that they have no programs in place to address the identified needs. A well-intended effort toward the physician is thus turned into a negative experience.

Database marketing.   Another form of direct marketing that deserves separate attention is database marketing. Database marketing has been pioneered in other industries (particularly financial services) and is a mechanism for extracting the maximum business out of existing customers. Database marketing involves developing an MCIF (marketing customer information file), which ideally includes records of all existing customers of the organization. This database is then used for followup sales, cross-selling, and as the basis for direct-mail programs.

Hospitals appear to be the best candidates for database marketing, although this approach could ultimately have applications for other providers. Ideally, the hospital's database should include records not only on all inpatients, but on any customer of the hospital. These could include people coming for outpatient tests, those patronizing the emergency room, clients of minor-emergency centers, or fitness program enrollees. The idea is to develop a comprehensive database as a basis for a variety of marketing efforts.

One approach identifies the constellation of services associated with any inpatient procedure. These services may precede hospitalization (and the procedure), occur during the procedure and subsequent hospital stay, or occur after hospitalization. The hospital identifies the total range of services associated with a particular inpatient procedure, determines whether or not all of the appropriate services are being provided (and charged), whether there are other services the hospital should offer, and whether some of these services are being lost to competitors.

Marketers can also identify customer segments that cut across product lines and specialties. These segments are categories of patients that require similar services and can be linked to other services across vertical hospital divisions. Customer segments can serve as the basis for marketing programs because they represent internally homogeneous segments with similar health care needs. Further, if linkages across specialties are identified, an episode occurring to a member of a segment can provide the basis for cross-selling other services.

Sequencing is a third approach that incorporates customer databases. Health care events affecting an individual (and a segment) often occur in sequence. If this sequence can be identified, any one event can serve as a predictor for other events. For example, the use of obstetrics is likely to trigger the use of pediatrics. When an event occurs to a member of a customer segment, this event triggers several other possibilities for cross-selling, repeat selling, and so forth.

Unlike other uses of the hospital MCIF, a fourth application focuses on potential customers rather than existing customers. The MCIF developed for other applications can also determine the "best" customers for various services. The characteristics of these customers can be used to clone similar customers from among both nonusers and competitors' customers. The "best" customers may be the heaviest users, the best payers, or the best candidates for related or followup services.

Developing and maintaining a database marketing program is no small undertaking. Unlike banking, where there is a long history of cross-selling, health care organizations have yet to develop the various linkages between services and customers. Developing this important component will require some time, as well as computer linkages of internal and external databases. In the meantime, existing customer databases can be used to do limited cross-selling and followup promotions.

Database marketing in health care has a different wrinkle from banks or other businesses. Some might question its usefulness because hospital visits are somewhat unpredictable and intermediaries such as physicians and insurers control much of the access. In actuality, health care episodes are surprisingly predictable if the population base is large enough to apply known rates. Proper market segmentation should allow the health care organization to predict the level and type of services required by specific segments. To the extent that the database includes physician referral information, it becomes a marketing tool for physicians as well.

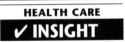

HEALTH CARE
✔ INSIGHT

The use of health care services may seem unpredictable, but it often follows a known sequence.

Finding the Customer: Desktop Market Analysis Systems

LOCATING PROSPECTS for any product is a challenging proposition, and it has been particularly challenging in health care, an industry without a history of market research. Efficiently identifying and targeting prospective customers is difficult enough with tried-and-proved research techniques and databases at the marketer's fingertips. Without these tools, the difficulties multiply.

Until the mid-1980s, health care marketers had few tools at their disposal; neither techniques nor databases were available. Then the first desktop market analysis system was introduced in 1985, and this led to a revolution in market research, especially for health care. For the first time, marketers could sit at their desks and, using one system, conduct a comprehensive market analysis. Not only were virtually all of the requisite databases and software packages at their fingertips, but they were magically interfaced within the desktop system. It was now possible to do comprehensive market research quickly and inexpensively. Most importantly, these systems did not just generate numbers—they offered solutions to market research problems and meaningful information for corporate decision makers.

Desktop market analysis systems can locate target populations, select sites, analyze the competition, plan direct-mail campaigns, and determine the appropriate media for a particular population segment. Depending on the databases available, internal patient data can be interfaced with externally generated information on demographics, economics and business, and consumer preferences.

Examples of desktop marketing applications in health care

▶

include the hospital seeking to introduce a new program, the nursing-home chain looking for additional sites, the health-insurance company expanding into new markets, the urgent-care chain seeking an additional location, and the physician group considering opening a second office.

Desktop market analysis systems have transformed marketing research from a slow plodding process of questionable accuracy to a highly scientific, accurate, and expeditious activity. Desktop analysis systems have made databases easily accessible and offer software packages that perform a number of sophisticated functions, such as simultaneously using multiple databases and creating "macros" to manipulate variables. Researchers can convert the results into reports, tables, graphics, and maps that depict the characteristics of the health care consumer and offer solutions to marketing problems.

Desktop market analysis systems effectively address most of the problems faced by market researchers operating in the health care environment. This is not to say that background information, forethought, and interpretive skills are not required; they certainly are. But it does mean that all the information for drawing conclusions is at your fingertips. In effect, in the hands of a knowledgeable analyst, the systems allow the questions to answer themselves.

Database marketing should grow in importance as hospitals move away from the inpatient mentality. After all, how many times can you sell a patient gallbladder surgery? Patients should be customers for a broad range of services, and as hospitals position themselves to take advantage of the outpatient market, this seems to be the way to go. The opportunity is not for repeat sales of acute-care services, but for capturing the related services associated with any illness episode.

The key attribute of all direct marketing is that it fosters ongoing communication with customers and potential customers. Unlike traditional media marketing, direct marketing keeps the health care organization close to the customer. It requires more in-depth knowledge of the customer while generating information on the customer that could not be developed in any other way.

Business-to-Business Marketing

In industries other than health care, business-to-business marketing has become increasingly competitive and is demanding ever more sophisticated techniques. Because of the manpower requirements involved in developing and maintaining corporate relationships, business-to-business marketing has to be highly efficient.

Hospitals and other health care providers are only now beginning to appreciate the usefulness of business-to-business marketing. Although historically, providers have dealt with a variety of organizations (and indeed, they themselves were operating as organizations), they saw themselves dealing mostly with the individual patient or physician. With the corporatization of health care, the hospital is less and less likely to deal with individual patients/customers. Today, the customer is much more likely to be an organization such as an employer, business coalition, or preferred-provider organization. This calls for a change in marketing approach.

Nonhospital care providers are seldom in a position to develop a sales force, and most, especially physicians, would find it distasteful to send sales representatives out to call on prospective corporate customers. However, they too must take some action in order to secure business that is becoming more and more corporate in nature. Physicians and certain other independent practitioners often rely on their community contacts for business-to-business marketing. Sports-medicine physicians may secure a position (perhaps without compensation) as a team physician in order to obtain the business generated by that group. A physician with an interest in occupational health may secure a position as a "company doctor" in order to capture the business generated by the employees.

Both hospitals and physicians need ways to deal with health maintenance organizations and preferred-provider organizations. Such organizations are looking for business relationships that meet the needs of their enrollees. In some cases, aggressive marketing is called for, such as when an employer is seeking to establish a primary-care network for its employees. In other cases, the main requirement of the provider is to astutely analyze managed-care contracts and make smart decisions regarding the relationships being negotiated. Above all, the provider needs to position itself beforehand as the type of organization with which the corporate purchaser of care would want to be associated.

Relationship Marketing

The shift from traditional marketing techniques to direct marketing, database marketing, and business-to-business marketing reflects the new wave for health care and other industries: relationship marketing. Despite the intimate nature of health services, many transactions have been treated as if they were one-time, impersonal events. Patients, physicians, employers, and others interacting with the health care system no longer accept this type of arrangement. They want a relationship that will be ongoing, work on a cooperative basis, and offer constant access. The key underlying all of these things is meaningful and ongoing communication and a commitment to service.

With health care, one is typically marketing intangibles, and this, of course, creates issues not important when marketing other products. Confidence and trust in health care providers is paramount. Trust is the basis for the doctor-patient relationship and should provide the foundation for any service delivery. Traditional marketing approaches that emphasize media do not develop this type of rapport.

Despite the fabled doctor-patient relationship, hospitals, physicians, and other health care providers have not done well in developing relationships. Health care events were seen as episodic. The "relationship" essentially began when the patient was admitted and ended when he was discharged (except of course for the ongoing negative financial relationship).

Like those marketing any service, health care marketers are really selling *solutions*. Solutions require ongoing attention and not one-shot responses. Media campaigns and impersonal service do not offer solutions and cannot provide the basis for relationship development. At the same time, consumers and payers alike are looking for "appropriate" services. They want a relationship that will channel patients into the right services rather than those that are the most profitable for the provider.

Hospitals and other providers have practical reasons to develop ongoing relationships. When figures were published concerning the lifetime "worth" of an individual's health care expenditures, some more progressive facilities began to take notice. It is one thing to capture a $5,000 hospital episode, but this pales in significance to the fact that the average consumer will spend between $150,000 and $200,000 on health care in his or her lifetime. This money goes somewhere, and hospitals began to realize it was not coming to them.

Similarly, physicians have seldom fully realized the potential "sales" from their existing patient populations. While it is true that physicians often have long-term and close relationships with some of their patients, how many other patients fail to show up for a routine exam or do not come back for a followup visit after treatment? If these were true relationships, the patients (and the money they would have spent) would not fall through the cracks.

Progressive health care organizations are beginning to realize that they want to acquire customers as well as maintain an ongoing relationship with them. Database marketing offers an approach that providers can use as a basis for relationship development. As the market for some services levels off, the pressure will mount to get the most out of existing customers. The only way to do this is through relationship development based on database marketing. In the future, it will not be sufficient to know who your customers are; you will have to know all about them.

Internal Marketing

One final consideration in developing a marketing program for a health care organization is internal marketing. Internal marketing involves organizing the operation to provide the best service possible. This means creating a climate that is totally customer-oriented. Every member of the organization must have this orientation, and managers must take responsibility for seeing that this happens.

Internal marketing also focuses on processing customers efficiently. It should ensure that procedures are set up for the benefit of the customer and not the staff. This begins with the initial call for an appointment, processing through registration, management of clinical assessment, subsequent billing, and followup contact.

Communication and coordination are critical factors in internal marketing. One of the most frequent reasons that problems in patient processing occur is a lack of communication. Health care organizations often create structural barriers to communication, and these must be addressed. Constant communication must occur throughout all levels of the organization.

Similarly, the uneven flow that often characterizes health care services creates barriers to coordination. Even if the left hand knows what the right hand is doing, their actions may not be well coordinated. Health professionals often accommodate themselves to this situation, but customers quickly become sensitive to the fact that their "case" is not being well managed. As corporate purchasers of care become more important, customers will have less tolerance for such failures. Strong internal marketing programs will be necessary to address these issues.

....

CHAPTER NINE

The Health Care Consumer and the Future

New Orientations for the 1990s

A number of trends that originated in the 1980s will fully develop during the 1990s. These trends will define the nature of health care into the next century. They will force health care organizations to change and adapt to the new environment. Health care organizations that survive will be those able to adjust to the changing world, and the winners among them will be those that position themselves to take advantage of these developments. Organizations that cannot adapt will be forced out of the market. The following developments will set the stage for health care during the rest of the 1990s.

During the 1990s, the transition from medical care to health care will be completed. The notion of a medically oriented, physician-dominated health care system will seem incredibly archaic. Health will involve more than freedom from illness and disability, and mean overall well-being, including physical, mental, and social factors. Health care will not be seen as something reserved for physicians, but as an endeavor in which a variety of parties, including patients and their families, should be involved. As a result of this broadening notion of health care, components that were marginal in the past, such as prevention, health education, and rehabilitation, will grow in importance. Various programs will begin to emphasize these types of services over acute care.

Health care providers will complete the transition from a product orientation to a service orientation. Steps taken in the 1980s will culminate in an approach that has providers behaving like other industries, where marketing is not a necessary evil but the engine that drives the train. Successful providers will reach the point where no decision will be made without testing the consumer waters. Services will be designed based on the needs (and wants) of consumers, not simply a reflection of what the hospital or clinic has always done. Responses from patients will drive changes made in existing services.

Providers will take the segmentation of health care to its fullest extent. Fewer and fewer services will be geared to the general public, as providers design products with distinct market segments in mind. Sophisticated database capabilities will match market segments to the service mix. Niche players will become more common, as the notion of comprehensive health care becomes less and less feasible. A possible negative side effect of this process is that providers will be able to carefully target the audiences they want, while avoiding the ones they do not want. This could mean that a larger number of patients will be thrown into limbo without easily accessible care.

New Organizational Structures

The developments of the 1990s will include some changes in the organizational structure of health care organizations. The 1980s saw innovations in health care financing that made parts of the system almost unrecognizable by the end of the decade. Comparable changes are anticipated for the 1990s, as market conditions require a rethinking of existing relationships and structures. The following examples provide an idea of what can be expected in the years to come.

Medical "malls" seem to be gaining interest and credibility. Medical malls bring together a variety of services under one roof, just as shopping malls do. They bring the concept of retailing (finally!) to health care. The idea is to establish a collection of outlets for goods and services that complement each other and, at the same time, offer comprehensive services. For the consumer, the medical mall offers the convenience of one-stop shopping. By consolidating services, a facility can provide services to areas where independent providers could not afford to. For example, few providers can afford to support a physical-therapy program on their own, but the combined resources and demand generated by a mall makes such a facility feasible. Furthermore, the combined resources allow for a better-furnished and more state-of-the-art facility.

For the developer, the mall concept creates a critical mass of services that provide more specialized diagnosis and treatment. Not only are economies of scale introduced, but carefully orchestrated internal referrals assure the success of all involved. Medical malls may have particular advantages for rural or semirural areas that can only support a limited level of services. A regional mall can draw from a large enough area to justify offering a greater number and perhaps higher quality of services.

The emphasis on relationships means that organizations will become more important than facilities. Today, employers, business coalitions, and other purchasers of care are less impressed with bricks and mortar than they are with the constellation of services. This trend portends "hospitals without walls." The hospital will be reformulated as a set of services and relationships rather than a collection of buildings.

Under one scenario, the only building that may be owned by the hospital organization is the facility for specialized inpatient care. The patient seeking services from the "hospital" may seek them from a variety of sources, many of which will be offered away from the hospital campus. Some, and perhaps most, services will not be offered by the hospital *per se*, but by organizations that have relationships with the hospital. The hospital without walls will offer services in a variety of settings, such as practitioners' offices, freestanding facilities, nonhealth care facilities such as community centers, and in the patient's home.

The developments carrying us into the 1990s will demand some innovative alliances. Despite the competition that has become so common in health care, cooperation is fostering arrangements between some strange bedfellows. Cooperative programs have already developed, with varying degrees of success, between hospitals and their medical staffs. In the 1990s we are likely to see alliances between providers, purchasers, and financers of care. These include hospitals and physicians on the provider side; employers, business coalitions, and health maintenance organizations on the purchaser side; and insurers and other third-party payers on the financer side. These alliances will establish mutually agreeable arrangements for buying, selling, and paying for health care.

The question facing providers of care as they move through the 1990s is what they should be and for whom. All providers must determine the mix of services they will offer and the audiences they will target. Hospitals in particular are already jockeying for position and reshuffling their service mixes. Even the most highly developed hospital systems cannot continue to be all things to all people. In effect, we can expect to see what might be called "controlled diversification."

Several developments are converging to reformulate health care as a "designed experience." According to the health care futurist, Russell Coile, the designed experience is badly needed to improve the deteriorating image of health care. Too often, the health care experience is a nightmare for consumers. Even if the clinical outcome is satisfactory, the long waits, the impersonal treatment, the cost, and just about everything else about the experience can be and often is negative.

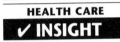

HEALTH CARE

✔ INSIGHT

The consumer's impression of the health care experience is paramount, and providers can design these experiences to appeal to the customer.

Although there are no adequate models as yet of a designed consumer experience in health care, some providers have taken steps in that direction. Birthing centers that have been designed with the users in mind, children's hospitals that make children *glad* to be there, and ambulatory-care centers that are set up as "comfort zones" begin to approach the designed experience. To really develop the concept, Coile points out, we must start from scratch in reconceptualizing health care, beginning with the needs and preferences of consumers.

Marketing Orientation of the 1990s

The challenges facing health care in the 1990s are expected to increase the interest in health care marketing. The industry must complete the conversion to a true service orientation, with much more of an "outreach" and marketing orientation than in the past. It is hard to predict exactly what the marketing-oriented hospitals or clinics of the future will be like, but there is a good chance that the successful ones will have most, if not all, of the following characteristics.

Service-oriented.   Providing service, in every sense of the word, will reflect the operational philosophy of the successful organization. In the 1980s, hospitals brought in consultants from the hospitality industry to teach them what they needed to know about serving patients and their families. (There is a note of irony here in that the words "hospital" and "hospitality" come from the same root word, and that hospitals were originally places for just that—hospitality. The early hospitals could do little to cure disease, so they strove to make their "guests" comfortable.) But health care providers will have to go well beyond lessons from the hotel industry to prosper in the 1990s. They will have to incorporate a service orientation that begins long before the patient is admitted to the hospital (if, in fact, he ever is!) and continues long after the hospital experience. Providers will move beyond providing service at the point of treatment and begin servicing a long-term relationship.

Consumer-driven.   The consumer will dictate virtually every aspect of the health care operation. Consumer preferences and needs will determine the constellation of services and products offered, the location of the facilities, the type of setting for service delivery, the types of practitioners used, and perhaps even the price. The health care organization may not be able to control all aspects of care (financing, for example), but the successful organizations will be those that design their operations for the benefit of consumers. They will listen to their existing customers and respond to their input. They will keep in touch with consumers who are not currently customers to determine their needs and how to best serve them. Marketing campaigns will reflect the needs of the consumer and not dwell on the merits of the organization.

Relationship-based.   The unit that measures the organization's activity will no longer be the admission, the outpatient visit, or the surgical procedure, but some indicator of the number and character of relationships that exist. Similarly, success will be measured by the number of industrial contracts that the organization maintains and the number of group purchasers and complementary health care providers with which it has formal relationships. Admissions, visits, and procedures will still be important, but they will be seen as a consequence of existing relationships and not vice versa. In the future, a relationship will not develop because a patient has been served by the organization, but the patient will be served by the organization because a relationship exists. The main goal of all health care organizations will thus be to develop, maintain, and enhance relationships in a variety of shapes and forms.

Service mix. As noted many times before, the health care provider of the 1990s cannot be all things to all people. The provider must decide what services to offer, how they will be offered, and how they will be marketed. The service mix will be variously influenced by the needs of the marketplace, the capabilities (and organizational relationships) of the provider, and the profitability of various services. This will result in the controlled diversification discussed above and may mean that many providers, in their service mix at least, look much different by the end of the 1990s than they did at the beginning.

Targeted audiences. The service mix will take care of "all things," while the targeted audience will take care of the "all people" component. The service mix established will not reflect the wishes of all consumers, only of those consumers the organization intends to target. Both mass marketing and image marketing will be "out," and carefully orchestrated target marketing will guide promotional campaigns.

Integrated marketing program. All components of the marketing effort must be coordinated and carefully interfaced. The phases of the process must be linked so that market research, product development, promotions, and followup evaluation flow smoothly. Similarly, providers must carefully coordinate efforts to determine product packaging, price, distribution channels, and marketing initiatives. Finally, activities must be coordinated across a variety of specialties, product lines, departments, and organizational functions if the process is to work. After all, the organization is now managing relationships, not individual treatment episodes. This calls for "seamless" marketing programs and a degree of integration undreamed of in the health care system of the past.

Areas to Target for the 1990s

The developments of the 1980s mean that the days of homogeneous health care are long gone. The challenge is to anticipate the types of services that will be in demand during the 1990s. Once identified, progressive health care organizations can position themselves to take advantage of the opportunities that the market is presenting. Some services can be anticipated without much debate such as services for the elderly, but beyond this, the health care marketer will have to become something of a forecaster. The following types of services will present significant opportunities during the 1990s.

Elder care.   Elder care is the consensus candidate for the remainder of the 1990s and into the next century. Even without changes in lifestyles, technology, practice patterns, or financing, the aging of the population clearly draws attention to services for the elderly. Even if the health of the elderly improves compared with past generations of elderly (as it seems to be doing), the numbers are still there. There are more elderly people in the U.S. today than at any time in the past, and the record will be broken every year for some time to come. The elderly require both a high level and a wide variety of services, and it is not necessary to belabor the point here. But marketers should be aware of the differences *among* the elderly and take those differences into consideration in developing services. They should also develop service with an eye toward the types of financing that will be available for elder care in the future.

Older adult services.   If there is a major category of services that will compete with elder care for attention during the 1990s, it is older-adult care. While it is true that older adults (i.e., those aged 45 to 64) do not require the same intensity of services as the elderly, in some ways they require a wider range. After age 45, chronic conditions become increasingly common, but acute conditions are still a consideration. Not only does physical impairment become a factor, but individuals in this cohort suffer from many conditions related to stress and psychological dysfunction. This is the age of mid-life crises, menopause, empty nests, loss of youth, and all those things that create anxiety for contemporary

Americans. What makes it so significant is that, in the 1990s, the huge baby-boom cohort is beginning to suffer from these conditions. They are also likely to react to aging much more aggressively than their predecessors. For example, procedures such as surgical reparation of vision loss should become a major business. This cohort is used to having things the way they want them, and they will have the money (and insurance) to demand a wide variety of services.

Home health.   Just as many Americans are returning to the home as the center of activity, so is health care. Most of the recent developments in health care point to a resurgence of traditional forms of home care and the development of innovative versions of it. Not only are patients themselves becoming more interested in receiving care in an informal, family-centered environment, but reimbursement mechanisms are encouraging home care as the low-cost alternative to institutionalized care. Technology has made forms of home care possible that would have been unthinkable in the past, and changing practice patterns are supporting this shift. The physician who makes house calls has re-emerged, and home births attended by midwives have gained some popularity. With the continued growth of the do-it-yourself health care market (*see below*), this trend should continue for some time.

Fitness and sports medicine.   The fitness craze that characterized the 1980s does not appear to be abating. More individuals from more market segments are participating in some type of fitness program. Many have always been active, while others are becoming fitness-conscious for the first time. This situation has created a boom in the demand for fitness programs and equipment. Who would have anticipated that aerobics training would become a major business? Consumers, particularly the fitness-oriented baby-boom cohort, have a lot of money to spend on memberships, lessons, and equipment. There is also a big market for health-oriented foods, as well as supplements and drugs that relate to fitness.

Increased fitness-related activities mean more sports-related health problems, especially among people who are not used to strenuous exercise. This should increase the demand for the services of orthopedic surgeons, physiatrists, rehabilitation counselors, and a variety of other health professionals in the sports medicine field.

Ethnic health care.   As the U.S. population becomes more racially and ethnically diverse, the demand for various types of services will change. Our system has come a long way from the traditional notion that the system represented the "right" way to provide health care, and that patients, regardless of ethnicity, nationality, or subculture, should conform to the demands of the system and be "good" patients. The diversification of the population creates both challenges and opportunities. Progressive health care organizations will view it as an opportunity to create customized services that cater to new target audiences. Many ethnic populations represent fertile areas for growth in health care demand, and many are becoming increasingly affluent. They see participation in this system as one of the perks of American society and are willing to pay for the services they receive.

Home diagnosis and treatment.   Although the health care system has never encouraged a do-it-yourself approach to health care, many consumers now serve as their own diagnosticians. An increasing number of tests are available for home diagnosis, and technological developments have made it possible for many individuals to monitor and treat their conditions at home. Home care addresses many of the current concerns of Americans—convenience, control, and cost-effectiveness. As with home health care, changes in financing mechanisms, consumers' preferences, and practice patterns are all pointing to growth in the demand for products that make safe and accurate home diagnosis and treatment feasible.

Preventive care.   The 1980s witnessed an incredible growth in the emphasis placed on prevention. Research revealed not only the health benefits of prevention, but the cost savings that widespread preventive care could accrue for the system and individual patients. The health care establishment has slowly come to accept prevention as an important component of care, and this process will no doubt be speeded along by insurers, employers, and other purchasers and financers of care who want the most bang for their health care buck. Individuals will seek practitioners with a prevention orientation, and corporate purchasers of care will insist that any services they purchase have an education component.

Rehabilitation.   As with preventive care, rehabilitation services have been a low priority in the U.S. health care system. Practitioners and insurers have considered it a necessary evil. As physical and mental impairment have become bigger issues in the health system, the need for more emphasis on rehabilitation has become obvious.

Not only has the number of disabled people increased, but we have become more sensitive to their needs. The 1980s witnessed the tragedy of millions of dollars spent on treatment and virtually nothing spent on rehabilitation, to the end that many of the treatment dollars were wasted. Rehabilitation is currently a growth area in health care and one that is well reimbursed. The maturing baby-boom cohort, with its insistence on having things in working order, can only fuel this demand.

Industrial health.   Industrial health programs became increasingly common during the 1980s, as employers and other purchasers of care tried to find ways to hold down costs. This was also a period of tighter health and safety controls, which resulted in a demand for consultation related to health issues within the industrial setting. Employers and insurers alike became sensitive to the counterproductive aspects of stress, emotional problems, and other dysfunctional conditions in the workplace. Industrial health opportunities can only increase as industry becomes more sensitive to its benefits, and as insurers, health maintenance organizations, and preferred-provider organizations offer incentives to maintain workplace health and safety.

Vanity market.   Although the demand for certain cosmetic procedures seems to have tapered off somewhat toward the end of the 1980s, this is probably only a temporary lull. In fact, it may be the calm before the storm. The aging baby-boom cohort may be the largest ever in both its demand for "vanity" services and its ability to pay for them. For a population segment that is used to controlling its destiny, it is a short step to taking advantage of the health care system to retain youth, vigor, and appearance. The variety of services and products available to serve this market will no doubt proliferate in the 1990s.

Perhaps the single most important factor for health care in the 1990s is the dominant setting for care. Ambulatory care settings will continue to be popular, and fewer services will be provided in an inpatient setting. This means that health care providers must position themselves to take advantage of this shift, and those who are heavily invested in inpatient services need to rethink their service mix.

As often noted, the developments underway are changing the nature of the health care system. Trends in technology, consumer preferences, provider practice patterns, and other factors are making the hospital admission an even rarer event than it already is. The hospital is being transformed from the court of first resort to the court of last resort. By the end of the decade, everything possible will be done to keep patients out of the hospital. If there is any one development of which the health care organization, and the marketer, should be aware, this is it.

SUGGESTED READINGS*

Anderson, Odin W. *Health in the United States*. Ann Arbor, MI: Health Administration Press, 1985.

Brown, Stephen W., and Andrew P. Morley, Jr. *Marketing Strategies for Physicians*. Oradell, NJ: Medical Economics, 1986.

Coile, Russell C., Jr. *The New Medicine: Reshaping Medical Practice and Health Care Management*. Rockville, MD: Aspen Publishers, 1990.

Francese, Peter, and Brad Edmondson. *Health Care Consumers*. Ithaca, NY: American Demographics, 1986.

Kotler, Philip, and Roberta Clarke. *Marketing for Health Care Organizations*. Englewood Cliffs, NJ: Prentice-Hall, 1987.

Mack, Ken E., and Philip A. Newbold. *Health Care Sales: New Strategies for Improving Quality, Client Relations, and Revenue*. San Francisco: Jossey-Bass, 1991.

Pol, Louis G., and Richard K. Thomas. *The Demography of Health and Health Care*. New York: Plenum, 1992.

Sullivan, Kevin W., and Meryl D. Luallin. *The Medical Marketer's Guide: Success Strategies for Group Practice Management*. Denver, CO: Medical Group Management Association, 1989.

Valentine, Stephen T., *Physician Bonding: Developing a Successful Hospital Program*. Rockville, MD: Aspen Publishers, 1990.

See appendix for additional sources.

APPENDIX
....
Sources of Data on Health Care Consumers

THE 1980S WITNESSED an explosion in the demand for data on health care consumers. The health care industry, which historically operated under a gentleman's agreement, suddenly found itself embroiled in cutthroat competition. There had been no need for market intelligence because the patients kept coming and the revenues were guaranteed. Almost overnight, hospital administrators and others seeking to understand health care consumer behavior began desperately seeking out market intelligence not only to succeed, but just to survive.

The sudden demand for data on health consumers was met by a dramatic increase in the supply of such data by government agencies. At the same time, commercial vendors began to fill some of the gaps left by government agencies and developed datasets that were not otherwise readily available.

The listings below provide an overview of health care data sources. It should be noted, however, that who the consumer is depends on one's perspective. Various parties might consider physicians, insurers, hospitals, or other health care entities the consumers of their goods and services. The references below focus on the end user of health care services—the patient. They are divided into publications and organizations, and also include private vendors that provide data on health care consumers. The lists are not exhaustive, but provide the basic resources for research on health care consumers.

PUBLICATIONS

Government References

Statistical Abstract of the United States. This annual publication of the U.S. Census Bureau is a general reference on a variety of topics. It includes a section on health data that focuses on health status, health facilities, health manpower, and health services utilization. It is a standard library reference book.

County and City Data Book. This biannual publication of the U.S. Census Bureau is a general reference on a variety of topics, with data for each city and county in the U.S. Data of interest to health care marketers include vital statistics, health facilities data, and health insurance data. The *County and City Data Book* is a standard library reference book.

Health, United States. This annual publication of the National Center for Health Statistics is a compendium of data from NCHS and a variety of other sources on health status, health services utilization, and health care consumer attitudes and knowledge. The book is available at libraries designated as repositories for federal publications and from the U.S. Government Printing Office and regional federal bookstores.

Mental Health, United States. Published approximately every four years by the National Institute of Mental Health, *Mental Health, United States* is the most comprehensive reference work on organizations providing mental health care, sources of funding for mental health care, and the characteristics of mental patients. The work is available at libraries designated as repositories for federal publications and from the U.S. Government Printing Office and regional federal bookstores.

Books

Almanac of Consumer Markets. Using data from the national Consumer Expenditure Survey, the *Almanac* (Margaret K.

Ambry, 1989) provides detailed statistics on health care spending by age cohort. In addition, it includes a variety of data on health status and health services utilization. *The Almanac* is available from American Demographics Books at (800) 828-1133.

The Health Care Book of Lists. *The Health Care Book of Lists* (Richard K. Thomas, et al.) is a compendium of data on health and health care. Drawing from a variety of sources, many of which are not generally known to the public, this reference work includes sections on health status, health services utilization, and other topics of interest to health care marketers. *The Health Care Book of Lists* is available from Paul M. Deutsch Press at (407) 895-3600.

Periodicals

Hospitals. Published twice a month, *Hospitals* is the official magazine of the American Hospital Association. Although geared to the needs of hospital administrators, the magazine often contains feature articles on health care consumer patterns and the results of surveys of health care consumers. *Hospitals* is usually available in medical-school libraries, although some general libraries may carry it.

Modern Healthcare. Published weekly, *Modern Healthcare* reports on the financial aspects of the health care industry. The magazine often contains feature articles on health care consumer patterns and the results of surveys of health care consumers. *Modern Healthcare* is usually available from medical-school libraries, although some general libraries may carry it.

American Demographics. Published monthly, *American Demographics* often includes articles related to health care consumers, as well as more general articles on consumer behavior with implications for health services utilization. This magazine is available from many libraries or by calling (800) 828-1133.

Journal of Health Care Marketing. Published quarterly by the health care division of the American Marketing Association, the *Journal of Health Care Marketing* carries articles, case studies, and how-to pieces related to health care consumers. The *Journal* is geared for marketing practitioners as well as academicians and is usually available from business-school libraries as well as some medical-school libraries. For additional information, contact Dr. Eric Berkowitz, Editor, at (413) 545-1203.

Advance Data. Published at regular intervals (with irregular special reports) by the National Center for Health Statistics, *Advance Data* reports findings from the National Health Interview Survey, the National Ambulatory Medical Care Survey, and the National Hospital Discharge Survey, among others. This series is available from libraries designated as repositories for federal publications and medical-school libraries. For additional information on this publication, contact NCHS at (301) 436-8500.

Vital and Health Statistics. Published at regular intervals (with irregular special reports) by the National Center for Health Statistics, *Vital and Health Statistics* reports on data on health status and vital statistics compiled by NCHS through its various reporting and survey programs.This series is available from libraries designated as repositories for federal publications and medical-school libraries. For additional information on this publication, contact NCHS at (301) 436-8500.

Health Care Financing Review. Published quarterly by the Health Care Financing Administration, *Health Care Financing Review* provides current data on the use and spending patterns of Medicare enrollees. Although a byproduct of the financial monitoring activities of the federal government, its reports provide useful insights into how the elderly are spending their health care dollars. The *Review* is available from most medical-school libraries and from many general libraries.

Newsletters

Health Care Competition Week. Published weekly, *HCCW* reports on trends that affect the competitive environment in health care. It often includes reports of studies on health care consumer behavior and predictions of future trends in the consumption of health services. *HCCW* is available from Capitol Publications, Alexandria, VA; telephone (703) 739-6444.

Marketing Women's Health Care.   Published quarterly, this newsletter reports on trends in the health care consumer behavior of women. Since women make a majority of the decisions related to health behavior, this information is critical. *Marketing Women's Health Care* is free and available from Dearing & Associates, Spokane, WA. The firm also performs custom research and marketing related to women's health care. Contact Mary Kelley at (800) 553-3344.

Medical Benefits.   Published biweekly, *Medical Benefits* focuses on trends in health care costs for employers and other entities that finance health care. It reports on factors influencing the health behavior of consumers and analyzes the manner in which the consumer's health care dollar is spent. Information is available from Panel Publishers, New York, NY; telephone (800) 562-1973.

Other Periodicals

Health Care Strategic Management

Health Marketing Quarterly

Healthcare Advertising Review

Healthcare Marketing Abstracts

Journal of Ambulatory Care Marketing

Marketing to Doctors

Medical Economics

Physician's Marketing

Senior Market Report

Social Science and Medicine

Strategic Health Care Marketing

ORGANIZATIONS AND VENDORS

National Center for Health Statistics. NCHS is the main federal clearinghouse for health-related data. The agency compiles data on vital statistics, conducts a variety of national surveys that involve health care consumer information, and disseminates registry and survey data in both printed and computerized form. In addition, NCHS has extensive unpublished data available. Its staff is available to provide information on any of the topics covered by its various data collection activities. Call (301) 436-8500, and your inquiry will be directed to the appropriate department.

National Research Corporation. NRC conducts nationwide health care consumer studies, as well as custom research activities. NRC also publishes a *Health Care Market Guide* for major cities and can customize reports for particular geographies. For additional information, contact Joyce Jensen at (402) 475-2525.

Professional Research Corporation. PRC performs nationwide health care consumer studies, in addition to its custom research activities. The firm conducts an annual national consumer trends study that examines patterns of health care use, consumer preferences, and consumer expenditure patterns. For additional information, contact Sheila Davis at (402) 592-5656.

Inforum, Inc. Inforum is a vendor of desktop analysis systems for the hospital industry. In addition to maintaining a variety of databases, Inforum conducts an annual nationwide survey of health care use trends, consumer preferences, and health spending patterns. Health consumer data can be obtained on a custom research basis or by accessing Inforum's existing databases. For additional information, contact Tim Garton at (800) 829-0600.

The Sachs Group. The Sachs Group is a vendor of desktop analysis systems for the health care industry. The firm also conducts an annual nationwide survey of health care consumers. Although access to the firm's databases is often restricted to users of the system, information is also available through custom research, data searches, and the firm's newsletter. For additional information, contact Linda Balkin at (708) 475-7526.

INDEX

Note: * indicates a diagram or chart

ABOUT THE AUTHOR

....

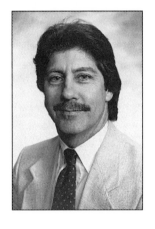

RICHARD K. THOMAS, Ph.D., is a life long resident of Memphis, Tennessee. Trained as a medical sociologist at Vanderbilt University, he has served as a senior research scientist at Baptist Memorial Hospital and has more than 15 years of experience in health services research, marketing and planning. He holds a faculty position at Memphis State University and teaches courses in sociology, health care administration, and marketing. Dr. Thomas has published books on the sociology of mental illness, health statistics, and the demographics of health care. He has published numerous magazine and journal articles and is on the editorial staff of the *Journal of Health Care Marketing*. He is an active consultant to hospitals, physician groups, and other health care organizations.

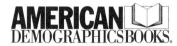

AMERICAN
DEMOGRAPHICS BOOKS.

Capturing Customers: *How to Target the Hottest Markets of the '90s*
Find out how to use consumer information to identify opportunities in nearly every market niche.

Beyond Mind Games: *The Marketing Power of Psychographics*
The first book that details what psychographics is, where it came from, and how you can use it.

Selling The Story: *The Layman's Guide to Collecting and Communicating Demographic Information*
A handbook offering a crash course in demography and solid instruction in writing about numbers. Learn how to use numbers carefully, how to avoid misusing them, and how to bring cold numbers to life by relating them to real people.

The Seasons of Business: *The Marketer's Guide to Consumer Behavior*
Learn which demographic groups are the principle players and which consumer concerns are most pressing in each marketing season.

Desktop Marketing: *Lessons from America's Best*
Dozens of case studies show you how top corporations in all types of industries use today's technology to find tomorrow's customers.

The Insider's Guide to Demographic Know-How: *How to Find, Analyze, and Use Information About Your Customers*
A comprehensive directory, explaining where to find the data you need, often at little or no cost.

The Almanac of Consumer Markets: *The Official Guide to the Demographics of American Consumers*
A clear, concise profile of the U.S. population that puts thousands of facts at your fingertips.